Statistics for Nursing

A PRACTICAL APPROACH

Elizabeth Heavey, PhD, RN, CNM

Assistant Professor of Nursing

SUNY College at Brockport

Brockport, New York

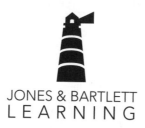

JONES & BARTLETT
LEARNING

World Headquarters
Jones & Bartlett Learning
40 Tall Pine Drive
Sudbury, MA 01776
978-443-5000
info@jblearning.com
www.jblearning.com

Jones & Bartlett Learning books and products are available through most bookstores and online booksellers. To contact Jones & Bartlett Learning directly, call 800-832-0034, fax 978-443-8000, or visit our website, www.jblearning.com.

Substantial discounts on bulk quantities of Jones & Bartlett Learning publications are available to corporations, professional associations, and other qualified organizations. For details and specific discount information, contact the special sales department at Jones & Bartlett Learning via the above contact information or send an email to specialsales@jblearning.com.

The author, editor, and publisher have made every effort to provide accurate information. However, they are not responsible for errors, omissions, or for any outcomes related to the use of the contents of this book and take no responsibility for the use of the products and procedures described. Treatments and side effects described in this book may not be applicable to all people; likewise, some people may require a dose or experience a side effect that is not described herein. Drugs and medical devices are discussed that may have limited availability controlled by the Food and Drug Administration (FDA) for use only in a research study or clinical trial. Research, clinical practice, and government regulations often change the accepted standard in this field. When consideration is being given to use of any drug in the clinical setting, the health care provider or reader is responsible for determining FDA status of the drug, reading the package insert, and reviewing prescribing information for the most up-to-date recommendations on dose, precautions, and contraindications, and determining the appropriate usage for the product. This is especially important in the case of drugs that are new or seldom used.

Production Credits

Publisher: Kevin Sullivan
Acquisitions Editor: Amy Sibley
Associate Editor: Patricia Donnelly
Editorial Assistant: Rachel Shuster
Senior Production Editor: Carolyn F. Rogers
Marketing Manager: Meagan Norlund
Associate Marketing Manager: Katie Hennessy

V.P., Manufacturing and Inventory Control: Therese Connell
Composition: Arlene Apone
Illustrations: diacriTech
Cover Design and Illustration: Scott Moden
Printing and Binding: Malloy, Inc.
Cover Printing: Malloy, Inc.

Library of Congress Cataloging-in-Publication Data
Heavey, Elizabeth.
  Statistics for nursing : a practical approach / Elizabeth Heavey.
      p. ; cm.
  Includes bibliographical references and index.
  ISBN 978-0-7637-7484-4 (pbk.)
  1. Nursing—Statistical methods. 2. Statistics. I. Title.
  [DNLM: 1. Statistics as Topic—Nurses' Instruction. 2. Nursing Research—methods—Nurses' Instruction. WA 950 H442s 2011]
  RT68.H43 2011
  610.73072'7—dc22
                                        2010017069

6048
Printed in the United States of America
15 14 13 12   10 9 8 7 6 5 4

Dedication

To Mr. Schmitt and the math teachers at Orchard Park High School . . . the skill and dedication you brought to the classroom every day laid the foundation I needed to tackle even more. You made this book possible.

And to my Mom and Dad, who made sure I didn't grow up being afraid of math—or anything else for that matter.

Contents

Chapter 3: *Descriptive Statistics, Probability, and Measures of Central Tendency* 29

Chapter 4: *Evaluating Your Measurement Tool* 47

Chapter 5: *Sampling Methods* 63

Foreword

Finally, a book that demystifies statistics!

The need for today's nurse to understand "patient-generated data" and to utilize information from statistical reports is greater than in any other period in the history of nursing. Today in nursing, the demands for accountability, achieving, and maintaining best practices and Magnet status are of paramount importance to making outcomes-based decisions. *Statistics for Nursing: A Practical Approach* is a remarkably timely book inasmuch as nurses are routinely responsible for planning related interventions to achieve the best possible clinical outcomes. Despite this demand, many nurses are reportedly intimidated by statistics.

This book is an excellent, much needed, user-friendly statistics book written by a nurse specifically for nurses. The book's emphasis is on enhancing understanding and facilitating the application of what has been learned. It streamlines more basic information while expanding the discussion of more complex, harder-to-grasp topics. The author's refreshing writing style, combined with case scenarios reflecting problems familiar to nursing, puts the reader immediately at ease. In the data-bound section of the book, which students typically find the most intimidating, the author demystifies the complexity of the formulas introduced, potentially capturing the interest and attention of the novice and expert alike.

Notably, the author does an outstanding job of assisting the nurse in selecting the most appropriate statistical measure to analyze data, whether the intent is to describe patient populations and outcomes or to draw inferences needed in planning or to better predict, prevent, and minimize workforce problems and patient complications. The book offers an abundance of useful case-based practical exercises designed to enhance the nurse's ability to interpret the data. These are indeed key strengths of the book.

Additional strengths of the book are the inclusion of a feature called "From the Statistician" (offering further clarity and expert opinions), a brief review of critical information at the end of each chapter, evidence-based research references for students seeking enrichment, and the integration of humor throughout the book, strategically placed to prevent student anxiety. The author coaches the student through the most difficult material in each chapter.

Finally, as a professor of research for over 20 years, my excitement about this new book is partly the result of its potential to provide students a smooth transition into research. When students are experiencing difficulty grasping the analyses section of my research course, I often refer them back to their statistics textbooks. Many express dismay at having continual difficulty comprehending material in their statistics book, despite having passed the course. I also find that students rarely, if ever, bring anything learned from their prerequisite statistics course to the research course, even when the course was completed only the prior semester. However, when discussing data analyses and findings, without question, students of the statistics course taught by the author of this book are more enthusiastic, can more easily apply what has been taught, and actively contribute to statistics-related course discussions. They are also better able to follow my rationales for why researchers selected a particular statistic to test hypotheses or to analyze data. In general, these students appear more capable of synthesizing research material than those taking traditional statistics courses.

I am convinced that this book, with its humor, clarity, and coaching, has the potential to leave students feeling that, with enough practice, they can become statistical geniuses. The book is exactly what the profession needs. It is indeed, the long awaited, academic solution to demystifying statistics.

Margie Lovett-Scott, EdD, RN, FNP-BC
Associate Professor of Nursing
Department of Nursing
The College at Brockport

Introduction

I am not a statistician. I am however, a nurse–midwife who likes to crunch numbers. (It must be a weird type of genetic mutation!) I combined these interests with a PhD in epidemiology and found a great niche for myself teaching at the college level and practicing with a great group of midwives one day a week. I love teaching and find that my students challenge me in ways I might never have anticipated, such as when they complained endlessly about not understanding the statistics class they had to take for the nursing major. The students arrived in my community health class convinced that they didn't understand and couldn't apply the statistical knowledge they had just learned. After going through several scenarios in class, it became apparent to me that the students had the capacity to do statistics, but anxiety and stress were getting in the way. When I explained the concepts in terms of nursing care, they grasped them and applied them in a whole different manner. That's when I decided that the trick to helping nurses learn statistics is to convince them they are not doing math; they are practicing nursing. Once I was able to convince my students that the skills we used for statistics were actually essential for nursing practice, the fear diminished, the anxiety decreased, and the learning began.

Nursing uses statistics regularly but we don't call it that. We call it quality improvement or risk assessment. We read and apply research and develop evidence-based protocols, most of which are reviewed with stringent statistical guidelines on a regular basis. All of these nursing skills involve statistics, and having a basic understanding of statistics makes for a better nurse. There is a strong history of using statistics to improve nursing care, dating all the way back to Florence Nightingale, who happens to be one of my personal public health heroes.

In the 1800s, she gathered and analyzed mortality rates for British soldiers at peacetime and compared them to civilian rates, discovering the soldiers were twice as likely to die from diseases or injuries as civilians. These were soldiers who were not fighting in a war and lived in England just like the civilians. In fact, she found that the peacetime mortality rates for the English soldiers were actually quite similar to the mortality rates of the soldiers stationed in Turkey fighting the Crimean war. She used this data and her statistical analysis to advocate for changes in public health policy and was known for her belief in gathering evidence to support the science involved in health care (Bostridge, 2008). Florence Nightingale paved the way for all nurses to incorporate statistics as an essential component of good nursing practice. Now we have to make sure we don't forget her message!

Because I believe so strongly that nurses need to understand statistics, I approached my department chair and the director of the RN-BSN program in which I teach and explained my experience with the stressed nursing students. I discussed how I thought our students could do much better at statistics if it was given in a class designed for nurses. I received what is the usual response from the wonderful group with whom I work—"Great idea! What do you need to make it happen?" And that is how I became a nurse who teaches statistics and gets the chance to talk about Florence Nightingale a lot.

While preparing for the class, I searched for a textbook. I found several excellent books designed for nurses at the graduate level but could not find an appropriate text specifically for nurses taking statistics at an undergraduate level. I used several texts and put together my own material for the pilot class, which the students were thrilled to take! I loved watching the nurses realize they could do statistics and that the field wasn't scary and foreign. It was a pleasure to see them work through clinical applications together and to have several come in to tell me that they were understanding things differently at work or had become involved in projects they had been too intimidated to join previously. During this time, Jones & Bartlett Learning contacted me about the text I was using. I explained that I had not found a text that fit well with what I was trying to do, and they sent me several to review. Again, no match. When I told them I was having no luck, they asked to see the material I was using for the class and then whether I would be interested in writing a book based on this curriculum. So that is how I ended up being a nurse who writes a statistics textbook! Who'd have thought!

I guess I never really foresaw how things would end up, but here we are and here you are. I hope you find the book helpful. I selected the topics for the book based on a review of the nursing research literature, in particular an article by Zellner, Boerst, and Tabb (2007), which identified the top ten statistical techniques used in nursing research. In addition to the topics they identified, I included Chapter 12, which is an overview of epidemiological statistical techniques. I have found, along with and Zellner, Boerst, and Tabb (2007), that these techniques are being used more and more in the public health nursing literature. Of course, I want you to be on the cutting edge of the most recently incorporated techniques in nursing research!

Keep in mind that this book is meant to be an introduction to some of the main concepts that nurses use in statistics. It is not designed to turn you into a mathematician or a statistician. You can use this course to pursue a path of statistical knowledge or as the basic course that lets you function safely in a clinical situation.

The text is designed so that each chapter builds on and reinforces previously taught material. You can skip the From the Statistician (FTS) sections and still have a very solid understanding of introductory statistics. Or, if you are more mathematically inclined, you can delve further into the topics utilizing the From the Statistician sections to really understand how the concepts were developed and relate. I keep most of the calculations and equations fairly basic (with the exception of those in the FTS portions) so that you can work your way through them with a calculator or a statistical computing package. If you would like to see how to use a statistical computing package to analyze data, a number of texts out there will help you, or you can go to the book website and run through a short tutorial. Statistical computing is a necessary next step if you wish to pursue statistics further, but it is used only minimally in this book (output is provided) so that you don't become overwhelmed right from the start. By the time you are done with the class, the prospect of using the computer to generate the statistical information you want won't be such a big deal. In fact, you may find that you want to do just that next!

The book ends with two appendices, both of which include a nursing research article. This is where you get to shine! After you have covered the material in the main text, you can use the appendices to review for a cumulative final or just to help you reinforce and retain the information you worked so hard to learn. Each appendix takes you through the article step by step and asks you to apply the information you covered in class to analyze and understand the content of the article. In addition, the website includes additional research articles and review questions you can use for review and practice. I encourage you to go through each of these as well as the review exercises in the book.

At the end of each chapter and on the website are review questions that give you even more opportunity to practice. The more you practice applying the material you learn, the clearer it will become and the more you will retain. I actually ask each of my students to master the material well enough to develop three test questions each week. (They need to produce and explain the answers as well.) I use the questions they come up with to assess what concepts the students understand and which concepts are still difficult for them. I also include questions that are very well done on the midterm and final for each class. Some of these questions are included in the test bank of questions that you can use for review or that your instructor can use for your exams. I always have at least one student who is completely surprised during an exam by seeing his or her own test question—which presumably is answered correctly!

During the writing of the book, I kept telling my brother, the statistician (probably the product of another genetic mutation!), that I wanted to limit the equations and calculations and emphasize the ideas nurses need to know. He wrote the FTS portions of the book and told me that doing statistics without a lot of equations and math is like trying to plant a garden without getting your hands dirty. That was a perfect example. I explained that this course is not meant to show anyone how to plant the garden; that is what upper-level statistics classes do. This course is to show students how to look at the garden, appreciate the different species, and recognize why one might grow better in the sun and another looks poor because it doesn't get enough shade. So here is your garden. You don't have to get muddy, but please do look at and enjoy all the different kinds of flowers!

—Beth

Acknowledgments

This book is the product of the combined effort of many individuals who were gracious enough to contribute their time, knowledge, and effort.

Brendan Heavey is the contributing author for all of the "From the Statistician" boxes in the text. Brendan has a statistical knowledge significantly beyond my own and spent many hours writing, rewriting, and explaining concepts to make sure my simplified explanations were technically correct. I am ever grateful not only for his statistical contributions to the text but also for his interest and support of the project from the early proposal days. He is an incredibly gifted human being. I am proud to call him my brother.

Dr. Linda Snell, Dr. Margie Lovett-Scott, and the department of nursing at SUNY Brockport recognized the need for a course that explained statistics in a way that nurses could relate to and understand. They supported my efforts in developing the first class we offered and later in formalizing the material so that nurses in other locations could benefit from the curriculum. I consider myself to be incredibly blessed to work with such an outstanding group of individuals who make going to work a rewarding and challenging experience every day.

Jessica Jackson, one of the best students I have had the opportunity to watch flourish, provided valuable feedback from a student perspective. Her review helped me determine when I had explained a concept well and also what needed revision.

The publishing team at Jones & Bartlett Learning, who saw the potential in this text before I did and helped make it happen.

As always, my heartfelt gratitude goes to my family and friends, who loved and supported me throughout this project. I would not be where I am today without all of you.

And to my children, Gabrielle and Nathaniel, being your Mama is by far my greatest joy. You put the meaning in everything I do.

Thank you all.

—*Beth*

Reviewers

The author and the publisher would like to thank the following individuals for reviewing the text:

Bakas, Tamilyn, DNS, RN, FAHA, FAAN, professor, Indiana University School of Nursing, Indianapolis, Indiana

Brooks, Evelyn, RN, PhD, Missouri Western State University, St. Joseph, Missouri

Hoisington, Denise, RN, MSN, PhD, Ferris State University, Big Rapids, Michigan

Letourneau, Nicole, PhD, RN, Canada Research Chair in Healthy Child Development, University of New Brunswick, Fredericton, New Brunswick

Pearsall, Catherine, PhD, FNP, CNE, St. Joseph's College, Patchogue, New York

Roberts, Beverly L., PhD, FAAN, FGSA, University of Florida, Gainesville, Florida

Ryan-Wenger, Nancy A., PhD, RN, CPNP, FAAN, Professor Emerita, College of Nursing, The Ohio State University, Director of Nursing Research, Nationwide Children's Hospital, Columbus, Ohio

Sorenson, Matthew R., PhD, RN, DePaul University, Department of Nursing, Chicago, Illinois

Worral, Priscilla Sandford, PhD, RN, Upstate Medical University, College of Nursing, Syracuse, New York

Introduction to Statistics and Levels of Measurement

How to figure things out.

Chapter 1

OBJECTIVES

By the end of this chapter students will be able to:

- State the question that statistics is always trying to answer.

- Define the empirical method.

- Compare quantitative and qualitative variables.

- Differentiate a population from a sample and a statistic from a parameter, giving an example of each.

- Explain the difference between an independent and dependent variable, citing examples of each.

- Identify continuous and categorical variables accurately.

- Distinguish the four levels of measurement and describe each.

- Apply several beginning-level statistical techniques to further develop understanding of the concepts discussed in this chapter.

KEY TERMS

Categorical variable
A variable that has a finite number of classification groups or categories, which are usually qualitative in nature.

Continuous variable
A variable that has an infinite number of potential values, with the value you measure falling somewhere on a continuum containing in-between values.

Dependent variable
The outcome variable or final result.

Empirical method
Gathering information through systematic observation and experimentation.

Estimate
A preliminary approximation.

Independent variable
A variable measured or controlled by the experimenter, the variable that is thought to affect the outcome.

Interval data
Data whose categories are exhaustive, exclusive, and rank ordered, with equally spaced intervals.

Nominal data
Data that indicates a difference only, with categories that are exhaustive and exclusive, but *not* rank ordered.

Ordinal data
Data whose categories are exhaustive, exclusive, and rank ordered.

Parameter
Descriptive result for the whole group.

Population
The whole group.

Probability
How likely it is that an outcome will occur.

Qualitative measures
A measure that describes or characterizes an attribute.

Quantitative measure
A measure that reflects a numeric amount.

Ratio data
Data whose categories are exhaustive, exclusive, and rank ordered with equally spaced intervals and a point at which the variable does not exist.

Sample
A group selected from the population.

Statistic
An estimate derived from a sample.

Variable
The changing characteristic being measured.

Introduction

So here you are. You've worked hard, been accepted into nursing school, and are ready to begin your studies. But wait! What do you mean you have to take statistics? Why does a nurse need to understand all those numbers and equations when you just want to help people?

Most nursing students experience a mild sense of panic when they discover they have to take statistics—or any other kind of math for that matter. That reaction is commonplace. Here is a calming thought to remember: *You already practice statistics, but you just don't know it.*

Statistics boils down to doing two things:

- Looking at data.
- Applying tests to find out either (a) that what you observe is what you expected or (b) that your observation differs enough from what you expected that you need to change your expectations.

You might be convinced that you don't use statistics in your life; so let me give you an example. New York State, where I live, has four seasons. The summer is usually June, July, and August. Fall is September, October, and November. Winter is December, January, and February. And that leaves March, April, and May for the spring. If you walk outside in July and find it to be 80° and humid, you would draw an unspoken conclusion that what you just observed is what you were expecting, and you would put on your sunglasses. However, what if you walk outside in January and find it to be 80° and humid? You would probably be startled, take off your overcoat and boots, and read up on global warming. The difference between the weather you expect in January and what you actually encounter is so different that you might need to change your expectations. You are already practicing statistics without knowing it!

Of course, that day in January might just be a fluke occurrence (a random event), and the temperature could be below freezing again the next day. That is why we need to use the **empirical method**, otherwise known as systematic observation and experimentation. The empirical method allows you to determine whether the temperature observed is *consistently* different from what you expect. To use the empirical method, you need to check the temperature on more than one day. So you might decide to mon-itor the temperature for the whole month of January to see whether readings are consistently different from what you expect. In this scenario, you would be using the empirical method to practice statistics!

Population Versus Sample

To answer questions in research, we need to set up a study of the concepts we're interested in and define multiple **variables**, that is, the changing characteristics being measured. In our example, the temperature is a variable, a measured characteristic. Each variable has an associated **probability** for each of its possible outcomes, that is, how likely is the outcome to occur. For example, how likely is it that the temperature will be below freezing as opposed to in the eighties? In your study, you recorded the temperature for only the month of January, and those readings make up a **sample** of all the days of the year. The manner in which you collect your sample is dependent on the purpose of your study. We will talk about this issue further in Chapter 5.

A sample is always a subset of a **population**, or an overall group (sometimes referred to as the reference population). In this case, our population includes all the days of the year, and the subset, or sample, is all the days in January. If you calculate the average temperature based on this sample data, you create what is called a **statistic**, which is an **estimate** generated from a sample.

A measured characteristic of a population is called a **parameter**. In our example, if you measured the temperature for the whole year and then calculated the average temperature, you would be determining a parameter. A really good way to remember the relationships among these four terms is with the following analogy: Statistic is to sample as parameter is to population.

Quantitative Versus Qualitative

While you are collecting the weather data, you may realize that the data can be recorded in several ways. You could write down the actual temperature on that day, which would be a **quantitative measurement**, or you could describe the day as "warm" or "cold," which would be a **qualitative measurement**. A numeric amount or measure is associated with quantitative measurement (such as 80°F), and qualitative measures describe or characterize things (such as, "So darn cold I can't feel my toes").

Be careful with this difference: You can easily get confused. *Qualitative variables do not contain quantity information, even if numbers are assigned. The assigned numbers have no quantitative information, rank, or distance.* For example, a survey question asks, "What color scrubs are you wearing?" and lists choices numbered 1–3. Even if you selected choice 2, neon orange, you do not necessarily have any more scrubs than someone who chooses 1, lime green (although both respondents may want to purchase new scrubs). Even though this qualitative variable has numbers assigned to it, the numbers simply help with coding. The variable is still qualitative.

Independent Versus Dependent Variables

Being as inquisitive as you are, you have probably asked yourself a number of times about a relationship you observe in your patients. For example, you notice that many supportive family members visit Sally Smith after her hip replacement recovery and that she is discharged three days after her surgery. Joanne Jones, on the other hand, has no visitors during her hip replacement recovery and is not discharged until day six. As an observant nurse

researcher, you have been wondering how variable x (the **independent variable**, which is measured or controlled by the experimenter) affects variable y (the **dependent variable**, or outcome variable). You wonder, does having family support (the independent variable) affect the duration of a hospital stay (the dependent, or outcome, variable)?

To answer this question, you create a study. Obviously, other factors might be involved as well, but in your experiment you are interested in how family support, the independent variable, impacts hospital stay, the dependent variable. If you are correct, then the duration of the hospital stay *depends* on family support. The independent variable can be the suspected causative agent, and the dependent variable is the measured outcome or effect.

Note: Additional criteria must be met to say a variable is causative; so I refer here only to the "suspected" causative agent. We will talk more about cause and effect later in the text.

Continuous Versus Categorical Variables

Some data have an infinite number of potential values, and the value you measure falls somewhere on a continuum containing in-between values. These values are called **continuous variables**. As a nurse, when you measure your patient's temperature, you are measuring a continuous variable. The reading could be 98° or 98.6° or 98.66666°. The infinite possibilities are all quantitative in nature. Actually the only limit to the measurement is the accuracy of the measuring device. If, for example, you have a thermometer that measures only in whole degrees, you will not have as much information as you would using a thermometer that measures to the one-thousandth of a degree.

FROM THE STATISTICIAN   BRENDAN HEAVEY

What Is a Statistic?

As a student of statistics, you will run into questions regarding parameters and statistics all the time. Determining the difference between the two can be difficult. To get a concrete idea of the difference, let's look at an example. According to the Bureau of Labor Statistics, registered nurses constitute the largest healthcare occupation, with 2.5 million jobs nationwide. Since this book is primarily designed for nursing students, let's use this number for our example.

Let's say you're a consultant working for a fledgling company that's planning to make scrubs for nurses. Let's call this company Carol's Nursing Scrubs, Inc. Scrubs at Carol's will come in small, medium, and large. The company will offer all kinds of styles and prints, but the underlying sizes are intended to remain the same. Carol just received her first bit of seed money to mass-produce 20,000 pairs of scrubs. Carol, an overly demanding boss, wants the medium-size scrubs to fit as many nurses nationwide as possible. To make that happen, she needs to know the average height and weight of nurses nationwide; so she has instructed you to conduct a nationwide poll. She thinks you should ask every nurse in the country his or her height and weight and then calculate the average of all the numbers you get.

Now, you are an intelligent, well-grounded employee who's in demand everywhere and working for Carol only because her health plan comes with a sweet gym membership and company car. So you realize it would be pretty difficult to set up a nationwide poll and ask all the nurses in the country for their height and weight. Even if you tried a mass mailing, the data returned to you would be filled with so many incompletes and errors that it wouldn't be trustworthy.

So what are you to do? Your first instinct might be to respond to your boss by saying, "Geez, Carol, that's so absurd and impossible I don't even know where I'd start" and then finish your day on the golf range. However, after this course you'll be not only a nurse, but a nurse with some training in statistics. You'll be able to deal with this situation in a more effective way. (Please excuse the weak dialog exchange here; there's a reason I'm not a screenwriter.)

Jenna the Statistical Nursing Guru (you):	Carol, I recommend we take a few *samples* of nurses nationwide and *survey* them rather than attempting to contact every nurse in the country. Then we could *estimate* the true average height and weight based on our samples.
Carol:	How would that work, Jenna?
Jenna:	Well, I'd go down to the University Hospital and poll 30 RNs on their height and weight. Then I'd go to the next state and do the same. My third and final sample would contain 30 RNs from a hospital in Springfield. I'd calculate the average from my total *sample* (90 RNs), which is a *statistic*, and use that to estimate the overall average in the United States, which is a *parameter* of the total *population*.
	You see, Carol, any time you calculate an estimate with data from a sample or list the data from the sample itself, you calculate a statistic. If you calculate an estimate from data in an entire population, you're calculating a parameter.

Continuous variables can be contrasted with **categorical variables,** sometimes called discrete variables, which have a finite number of classification groups, or categories, that are usually qualitative in nature. For example, as part of your research you may need to collect information about your patients' racial background. The choices available are African American, Native American, Caucasian, Asian, Latino, mixed race, and other. Race is an example of a categorical variable, a measurement that is restricted to a specific value and does not have any fractional or in-between values.

Levels of Measurement

Let's say your interest in the relationship between family support (the independent variable) and duration of stay (the dependent variable) is extensive enough that you apply for a program at your hospital that includes a small research fellowship. You win the fellowship and proceed to collect data about each patient admitted to your orthopedic unit for hip replacement over a three-month period. The study protocol calls for you to complete the usual admission forms and then for patients to complete a short survey about perceived family support. After your institutional review board approves your study, you begin. The level of measurement of your data determines what type of analysis you are able to perform in your study so let's look at the different types and what makes each level unique. Your first question asks the patient's gender: male or female. The data you gather for this question is an example of **nominal data**; it simply indicates a difference between the two answers. One is neither greater nor less than the other, and they are not in any particular order. Also, the categories are exclusive and exhaustive; that is, the patient cannot answer "both" or "neither."

You then ask the patient to rate his or her family support level as low, medium, or high. This question is an example of **ordinal data.** Ordinal data must be exhaustive and exclusive, just like nominal data, but the answers are also rank ordered. With rank-ordered data, each observation/ category is higher or lower or better or worse than another, but you do not know the level of difference between the observations/categories. In this example, a high level of family support indicates a greater quantity of the variable in question than low levels of family support.

A routine part of admitting each patient also includes a baseline set of vital signs. So one of the vital signs you check is each patient's temperature. Temperature is an example of **interval data**, which is exhaustive, exclusive, and rank ordered and which has numerically equal intervals. In this example, the interval is a degree of Fahrenheit.

After assessing each patient's temperature, you go on to take each patient's blood pressure. Blood pressure is an example of **ratio data**, which is exhaustive, exclusive, rank ordered with equal intervals *and* a point at which the variable is absent. (If the blood pressure reading is "absent" in any of your patients right now, please stop reading and begin CPR!)

Ratio data is the highest level of measurement you can collect and gives you the greatest number of options for data analysis, but not all variables can be measured at this level. As a general rule of thumb, always collect the highest-level data you can for all your variables, especially your dependent variable. In your study of how family support (the independent variable) impacts the duration of hospital stay (the dependent variable), you could have measured the length of hospital stay as short, medium, or long (ordinal) or in actual days (the interval/ratio level). Obviously, the actual number of days gives you a higher level of measurement.

Note: A dependent variable with a higher level of measurement allows for a more robust data analysis. Collect the highest level you can!

Summary

Talk about exhausting! You survived Chapter 1! So let's wrap it up here. Statistics really boils down to asking:

- Is what you observe what you expect?
- Or using the empirical method, have you determined that what you observe is different enough from what you would expect that you need to change your expectations?

Using qualitative (descriptive) and quantitative (numeric) variables, you can assess the impact of independent variables on dependent (outcome) variables. Always collect the highest level of measurement possible, especially for your dependent variable. Doing so gives you the widest range of analysis options when you are ready to "crunch the numbers."

If you understand these concepts, you are ready to move on to the review exercises. If you are still struggling, don't despair. These concepts sometimes take a while to absorb. Read the review questions and then the chapter again, and slowly start to look at the review questions. You will get the hang of statistics; sometimes you just need practice. My students frequently look at me as though I am an alien when I tell them that by the end of the course this chapter will seem really simple. You may not believe it either. However, as you develop your understanding and apply these concepts, they will become clearer, and you too will look back in amazement. You are a statistical genius in the making!

CHAPTER 1 REVIEW QUESTIONS

1. A researcher asks hospitalized individuals about their comfort in a new type of hospital gown. This is an example of what type of data?
   a. ratio
   b. independent
   c. quantitative
   d. qualitative

2. If a researcher is examining how exposure to cigarette ads affects smoking behavior, cigarette ads are what type of variable?
   a. qualitative
   b. quantitative
   c. dependent
   d. independent

(continues)

3. A nurse practitioner measures how many times per minute a heart beats when an individual is at rest versus when running. She is measuring the heart beat at what level of measurement?

   a. interval/ratio

   b. nominal

   c. independent

   d. ordinal

4. If a researcher is examining how exposure to cigarette ads affects smoking behavior, smoking behavior is what type of variable?

   a. ratio

   b. independent

   c. dependent

   d. nominal

5. The research nurse is coding adults according to size. A person with a below-average BMI is coded a 1, average is 2, and above-average is 3. What level of measurement is this?

   a. nominal

   b. ratio

   c. ordinal

   d. interval

6. You are asked to design a study measuring how nutritional status is related to serum lead levels in children. You assess calcium and fat intake, as well as serum lead levels in a sample of 30 2-year-olds. Lead levels are measured in micrograms per deciliter (mcg/dL). For example, one child had a lead level of 17 mcg/dL. This is an example of what type of variable?

   a. quantitative

   b. qualitative

   c. independent

   d. nominal

Questions 7–9: You are asked to design a study to examine the relationship between pre-operative blood pressure and postoperative hematocrit.

7. What is your independent variable?

8. What is your dependent variable?

   _____

9. How will you measure each, and what level of measurement is this?

   _____

   _____

Questions 10–13: You are later asked to do a follow-up study to see whether requiring a postoperative blood transfusion impacted postoperative rates of poor mental health, specifically depression.

10. What is your independent variable?

    _____

11. What is your dependent variable?

    _____

12. How will you measure them and why?

    _____

    _____

13. Is your dependent variable measured at the highest level? If not why not?

    _____

    _____

Questions 14–16: You decide to measure depression on the following scale: 1 = low, 2 = moderate, 3 = high.

14. This is what level of measurement?

    _____

15. How could this measure be improved?

    _____

16. Why might you want to improve it?

    _____

17. You decide to measure postoperative hematocrit by serum levels. Is this a quantitative or qualitative measurement?

    _____

(continues)

18. You discover that all but those with the lowest hematocrits had higher levels of depression after their surgery and transfusion. Why might the group that had the most critical need for the transfusions not have the subsequent depression associated with this result in the rest of your sample?

_____

Questions 19–25: Serum lead levels below 10 mcg/dL in childhood are associated with lower IQ, whereas levels above 10 mcg/dL are related to hyperactivity, aggression, poor growth, diminished academic performance, increased delinquency, seizures, and even death. The neurological damage that occurs cannot be reversed, even once exposure is stopped.

19. You have been asked to follow up in your community and determine what outcomes are associated with lead exposure in children. List three dependent variables for your study and how you will measure them.

_____

_____

_____

20. What level of measurement are your dependent variables? Are they continuous or categorical?

_____

21. Can you increase the level of measurement for any of them?

_____

22. If you are looking at what outcomes are associated with lead exposure in children, what is your independent variable?

_____

23. Why might it be difficult to measure?

_____

24. Describe how it could be measured quantitatively or qualitatively.

_____

_____

25. Which do you prefer? Why?

_____

_____

Use your computer to practice these applications. The companion website for this book has a computer-based application example (using SPSS, an IBM company[1]) for this material. Check it out!

[1]SPSS was acquired by IBM in October 2009.

| Analyze | Graphs | Utilities | Add-ons | Window | Help |

Reports ▶

Descriptive Statistics ▶   Frequencies...

Tables ▶   Descriptives...

Compare Means ▶

ANSWERS TO CHAPTER 1 REVIEW QUESTIONS

1. D

3. A

5. C

7. Preoperative blood pressure

9. Answers may vary—actual blood pressure-ratio, lab reported hematocrit-ratio, and so on.

11. Depression

13. Answers may vary.

15. Use of interval data, such as Beck's depression scale

17. Quantitative

19. Answers may vary, including IQ, school enrollment, crime, pregnancy, hematocrit, learning disabilities, growth, hearing, and behavior.

21. Answers will vary.

23. Answers may vary and include, "It requires a blood draw," "There are different testing mechanisms," "The level may change depending on when the exposure occurred and the time that has lapsed since then," "Levels may differ from fingersticks versus serum draws."

25. Answers will vary.

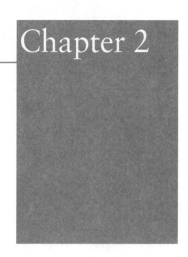

Presenting Data

Will my audience be able to see what the data is saying?

OBJECTIVES

By the end of this chapter students will be able to:

- Describe a frequency distribution.
- Identify situations in which a grouped frequency distribution is helpful.
- Calculate a percentage.
- Determine the percentile rank of an observation.
- Calculate the cumulative frequency and the cumulative percentages for a group of data.
- Develop a frequency distribution.
- Identify the best visual representation for various types of data.

KEY TERMS

Bar chart
A chart that has the nominal variable on the horizontal axis and the frequency of the response on the vertical axis, with spaces between the bars on the horizontal axis.

Cumulative frequency
The number of observations with a value less than the maximum value of the variable interval.

Cumulative percentage
The percentage of observations with a value less than the maximum value of the variable interval.

Frequency distribution
A summary of the numerical counts of the values or categories of a measurement.

Grouped frequency
A frequency distribution with distinct intervals or groups created to simplify the information.

Histogram
A chart that usually has an ordinal variable on the horizontal axis and the frequency of the response on the vertical axis, with no spaces between the columns on the horizontal axis.

Line graph
A chart in which the horizontal axis shows the passage of time and the vertical axis marks the value of the variable at that particular time.

Outlier
An extreme value of a variable, outside the expected range.

Percentage
A portion of the whole.

Percentile rank
The percentage of observations below a particular value.

Percentiles
Divides the data set into 100 equal portions.

Quartiles
Divides the data set into four equal portions, with the first quartile the 25th percentile, the second quartile the 50th percentile, the third quartile the 75th percentile.

Scatterplot
A chart in which each point represents the measurement of one subject in terms of two variables.

Frequency Distributions

Once you have designed a study and collected data, the next step is to decide how to present the assembled data. You have several options for doing so. The first and most common choice is a **frequency distribution**, which shows the fre-quency of each measure of a variable. A frequency distribution is created by gathering all the responses collected from a sample of vari-ables into a table (see Figure 2-1). The first col-umn of the frequency distribution in Figure 2-1 shows the number of days spent postoperatively in the hospital (your dependent variable from

Chapter 1), sorted from the shortest stay to the longest. The second column shows how frequently that length of stay was needed, that is, the number of patients who spent each number of postoperative days in the hospital. These two columns display the total numeric value of the variable of interest (in this case, the dependent variable, days spent in the hospital), usually ordered from the lowest to the highest. You can see the frequency of each level of the variable and its spread (distribution). The frequency distribution table presents a big-picture view of your data.

To augment a frequency distribution table and really impress your colleagues, you can add a **cumulative frequency** column, which simply lists the number of observations with a value less than the maximum value of the variable interval. For example, in the third column of Figure 2-1, second row, the number 9 means that 9 patients have stayed either 2 or 3 days postop in the hospital. The number 9 is the cumulative frequency for the first two intervals (2 and 3 days) of the variable. Let's say you are putting together an in-service presentation and decide to collect data from a set of patients on how many postop days they spent in the hospi-

tal. You find that 9 patients were discharged on day three or earlier; that total includes all the patients who stayed for 2 or 3 days. It is a cumulative frequency.

Now your nurse manager approaches you in a panic because the accreditation agency is coming next week and she needs to know how many patients were discharged after more than four days of recovery? The best way to visually answer that question is to create a new table that includes **grouped frequencies**, which is a frequency distribution with distinct intervals or groups created to simplify the information. In Figure 2-2, the values of the frequency distribution in Figure 2-1 have been collected into two groups: (1) patients who spent 4 days or fewer in postop and (2) those who spent 5 days or more. Grouped frequencies are typically used when working with a lot of data and an entire frequency distribution is simply too large to be meaningful.

Unfortunately, when data is grouped, some information is lost. For example, how many patients in Figure 2-2 stayed only 2 days? The answer is not discernible from this table. This is the first drawback to be aware of when using grouped frequencies; you can lose a lot

Figure 2-1 Frequency Distribution Table for the Length of the Hospital Stay.

Days Spent in the Hospital Postop	Number of Patients Who Stayed This Long (Frequency)	Number of Patients Who Stayed This Long or Less (Cumulative Frequency)
2	2	2
3	7	9
4	23	32
5	14	46
6	4	50

Figure 2-2 Frequency Distribution Table for the Length of Hospital Stay Using Grouped Frequencies.

Days Spent in the Hospital Postop	Numbers of Patients Who Stayed This Long (Frequency)
≤ 4 days	32
5 or more days	18

Figure 2-3 Calculating a Percentage.

$$\frac{18}{50} = 0.36 \times 100 = 36\%$$

of information when you convert your data into groups, especially if you use large intervals. You can even make the intervals so large that they are meaningless. In our example, if one interval were more than 7 days and the other were less than 7 days, the table in Figure 2-2 would not be very useful anymore because all the patients in the study were discharged by day seven. On the other hand, make sure not to make the intervals too small or your grouped frequency won't have any benefit over a standard frequency distribution.

Let's return to our example of the poor nurse manager who needed to get ready for the accreditation agency visit. After retabulating the data as shown in Figure 2-2, you can calmly go into her office and tell her that, during the period of time in your study, 18 patients were discharged after more than four days of recovery.

Percentages

A **percentage** is a part of the whole. To calculate a percentage, divide the partial number of items by the total number of items and then multiply that quantity by 100. For example, what if that same nurse manager asked you, "What percentage of our patients do those 18

represent?" You could do the simple calculation shown in Figure 2-3. In this example, the number of patients of interest (those who were discharged after day four) is 18. The total number of patients studied is 50. (See the last line of the third column in Figure 2-1.) The first step in our calculation is 18 ÷ 50. This division results in 0.36, which is then multiplied by 100 to get a percentage of 36%.

Exam scores are a classic example of percentages. If you take an exam with 30 questions and get 27 correct, what is your overall score? In this case, divide 27 by 30 and then multiply by 100 to get 90%.

A statistics concept commonly associated with percentages is **cumulative percentage**, which is the percentage of observations with a value less than the maximum value of the variable interval. The idea is the same as cumulative frequency, but expressed as a percentage. See the rightmost column of the table in Figure 2-4 for an example. The last column shows the conversion of each cumulative frequency (from Figure 2-1) into a cumulative percentage.

That column shows what percentage of patients had a hospital stay of less than or equal to the number of days listed in that row. For example, 18% of patients had a hospital stay of less than or equal to three days, and all of the patients (100%) were discharged on or before day six (see the last line of the last column).

Percentages are also closely related to percentiles, which are explained in the next "From the Statistician."

Figure 2-4 Cumulative Percentage Table for Length of Hospital Stay.

Days Spent in the Hospital Postop	Number of Patients Who Stayed This Long	Cumulative Frequency	Cumulative Percentage
2	2	2	$2/50 = 0.04 \times 100 = 4\%$
3	7	9	$9/50 = 0.18 \times 100 = 18\%$
4	23	32	$32/50 = 0.64 \times 100 = 64\%$
5	14	46	$46/50 = 0.92 \times 100 = 92\%$
6	4	50	$50/50 = 1.0 \times 100 = 100\%$

FROM THE STATISTICIAN   BRENDAN HEAVEY

Quantiles, Quartiles, and Percentiles—Oh My!

These three terms cause a lot of people grief because they are so closely related. So let's break them down a little. Using quantiles is just like dividing a data set into different portions or bins. Two special cases of quantiles are percentiles and quartiles.

- **Percentiles** divide a data set into 100 equal portions. You see this concept used with body mass index (BMI). If a patient's BMI is in the 90th percentile, then 90% of the BMIs in the reference population used to develop the distribution were at or below this patient's BMI. Put another way, this patient's BMI is in the top 10% of the reference population.
- **Quartiles** divide a data set into four equal parts. For example, suppose your nursing manager wants to hire only students who finished in the top quarter of the class on a particular exam. She would calculate the third quartile and select all the scores above it. Since your score would clearly be near the top, she would then rush to your school and attempt to woo you with new scrubs and tuition benefits!

How would the nursing manager compute a percentile? Let's say a sample of 331 nurses at Massachusetts General Hospital were asked how many patients they see on average each shift. The results of this survey are shown in Figure 2-5. A nice formula to find percentiles in the ordered data set is shown in Figure 2-6. For instance, based on the ordered data set in Figure 2-5, we apply the formula as shown in Figure 2-7 to find what is called the median, or the middle observation when the observations are lined up in rank order (least to greatest). The median is also the 50th percentile. Therefore, our median is our 166th observation. Using Figure 2-5, we can see that the nurse who was observation #166 saw 16 patients.

Because the total sample is 331, the middle observation is the 166th observation. If you add all the nurses who saw fewer than 16 patients, you find that 155 of them reported seeing fewer than 16

(continues)

FROM THE STATISTICIAN   BRENDAN HEAVEY

patients and 22 others saw 16 patients. After lining up the observations in rank order, the 166th observation falls into the group who reported seeing 16 patients; that group is the median. Using the formula takes less time than the old-fashioned way: adding them up.

You can also check yourself by looking at the cumulative relative frequency column. The median should be where the midpoint is. In Figure 2-5, look at the row for 15 patients, and see the corresponding cumulative frequency percentage; 47% of the nurses reported seeing 15 or fewer patients. Look at the next line, for 16 patients; 53% of the nurses reported seeing 16 or fewer patients. Therefore, the 50th percentile is above 15 and less than or equal to 16. Since we cannot split a patient into parts (at least for statistical purposes!), the median number of patients is 16.

Figure 2-5 Frequency Table for Sample of 331 Nurses at Massachusetts General Hospital.

Number of Patients	Number of Nurses	Relative Frequency (%)	Cumulative Relative Frequency (%)	Number of Patients	Number of Nurses	Relative Frequency (%)	Cumulative Relative Frequency (%)
1	0	0.00	0.00	16	22	0.07	0.53
2	0	0.00	0.00	17	20	0.06	0.60
3	2	0.01	0.01	18	19	0.06	0.65
4	3	0.01	0.02	19	18	0.05	0.71
5	5	0.02	0.03	20	19	0.06	0.76
6	8	0.02	0.05	21	17	0.05	0.82
7	8	0.02	0.08	22	15	0.05	0.86
8	9	0.03	0.11	23	12	0.04	0.90
9	9	0.03	0.13	24	8	0.02	0.92
10	12	0.04	0.17	25	9	0.03	0.95
11	14	0.04	0.21	26	5	0.02	0.96
12	18	0.05	0.27	27	5	0.02	0.98
13	22	0.07	0.33	28	3	0.01	0.99
14	23	0.07	0.40	29	3	0.01	1.00
15	22	0.07	0.47	30	1	0.00	1.00

331 nurses at Massachusetts General Hospital were asked how many patients they saw on their shifts that night. Results are displayed. Relative frequencies are computed by dividing the number of nurses who saw each number of patients by the total number of nurses (331). Each cumulative relative frequency is the result of adding the previous row's relative frequency to its cumulative relative frequency, so in essence cumulative relative frequency is an accumulation of relative frequency.

Figure 2-6 Formula for Calculating Percentiles in an Ordered Data Set.

$$P_{obs}^{th} = (n + 1) \times \frac{y}{100}$$

where

P_{obs}^{th} = the number of the observation at the percentile for which you are looking

n = the number of observations in your data set

y = the percentile you're looking for

Figure 2-7 Equation for the Massachusetts General Sample.

$$P_{obs}^{th} = (331 + 1) \times \frac{50}{100} = 166$$

Percentages are also related to the concept of **percentile rank** of a score, which is the percentage of observations lower than that score in a frequency distribution. For example, if your test score is greater than 75% of all the scores for the class, it is at the 75th percentile.

Bar Charts

Remember nominal categorical data (the categorical data that shows only a difference and is not rank ordered)? A **bar chart** is one way to display this type of data. A common way to set up the bar chart is to line up the responses for the nominal variable along the horizontal axis and place the frequencies of the responses on the vertical axis. Bar charts are typically used for nominal categorical data with spaces between the bars because each answer is distinct and in no particular order. For example, if you collected data about the marital status of fellow nurses on your unit, you might find data like in Figure 2-8. A quick look at the bar chart makes it apparent that most of the nurses working on this unit are single. The bar chart gives you a good visual representation of nominal categorical data.

Bar charts can be used for ordinal data as well, but then the bars should follow the rank order of the variable categories.

Histograms

Histograms are a type of bar chart. Histograms often have no spaces between the bars because these charts are most frequently used to display either ordinal data or continuous data. (Remember, ordinal data has categories that show a ranked difference; continuous data has an infinite number of possible in-between measures.) For example, pain may be rated as mild, moderate, or severe.

Figure 2-8 Bar Chart for Marital Status.

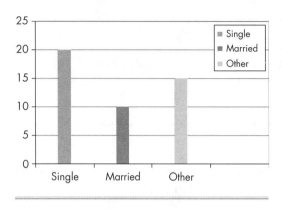

Presenting these types of data in a histogram shows how frequently each response is selected and allows for visual comparison of the different levels. In Figure 2-9, 11 patients were interviewed 12 hours postop from abdominal surgery. Six rated their pain as severe, four

Figure 2-9 Histogram for Pain Level.

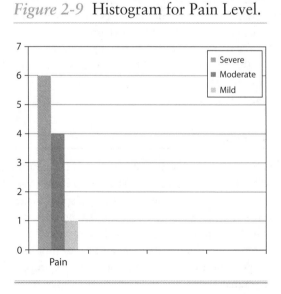

stated it was moderate, and one felt it was only mild (he had just had his pain meds!). The lack of spaces between the bars in the histogram reinforces the idea that these responses are on a continuum and that the order is illustrated on that continuum.

Looking at this histogram gives you a big-picture idea of the pain these patients experienced. In this case, the histogram seems to indicate that many postop patients report the first 24 hours as being very painful. So the next time you orient a new nurse, you might remember to point out how important it is to make sure patients have their pain medicine ordered and administered on time immediately after surgery. The chart also visually displays that many patients may not be getting adequate pain medication because so many report severe pain. After collecting this data, you may decide to review the unit protocols for pain management.

Line Graphs

Continuous variables that change over time are frequently best illustrated in a **line graph**. The horizontal axis shows the passage of time, and the vertical axis marks the value of the variable over time. For example, the data from the cumulative frequency example about days of hospitalization is illustrated in Figure 2-10. The chart shows that most of the patients needed to stay four days postop before going home. You might want to compare this line graph to another after you institute an early mobilization plan with your surgical patients to see whether the length of hospitalization has changed.

Scatterplots

Scatterplots are a little different than the previously discussed graphs in that each point represents how one subject relates to two variables.

Figure 2-10 Line Graph for Length of Hospitalization.

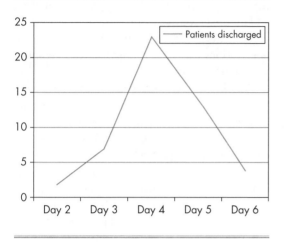

For example, Figure 2-11 shows a scatterplot of height in inches and weight in pounds for a group of 8 kindergartners. Each square on the scatterplot represents one student. The horizon-

Figure 2-11 Scatterplot for Student Height (x axis) and Weight (y axis).

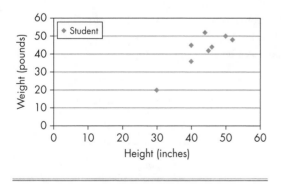

tal axis displays that student's height, and the vertical axis displays his weight. You can see from the direction of the plotted points that, as students get taller, they usually get heavier as well; that's the relationship between the two variables. When points are close together or seem to follow a line closely, the relationship between the variables on the horizontal and vertical axis are relatively strong.

When you look at a scatterplot, note the general trend. In this example, the plotted points start low on the left-hand side and move up as they progress toward the right side. This pattern indicates a *positive relationship* between height and weight (in other words, they usually move in the same direction—when height increases, weight usually does too). If the plotted points were to start in the upper left corner and slope down to the right, the pattern would indicate a *negative relationship* between the two variables (such as exercise and weight—when exercise is increased, weight usually decreases).

Scatterplots also give nurses a chance to look for **outliers,** or data that is outside the expected relationship. In Figure 2-11, the student who is only 30 inches and 20 pounds clearly stands out from the rest of the group. Perhaps the child is just extremely small, or there may have been an error in measurement, recording, or data entry. If there are a lot of outliers, a nurse may decide either that further investigation is needed to ensure accuracy or that the outliers may actually represent the children the study is designed to identify. One example of this technique is the use of growth charts. In almost all cases when children make pediatric visits, nurses plot the childrens' heights and weights on a growth chart. This is one example of using a scatterplot to look for outliers. If a child isn't growing properly, recognizing the growth pattern as an outlier is one way to identify a child who needs intervention.

Summary

This chapter added quite a bit more information. So let's review and make sure you are really comfortable before you go on. Frequently, researchers put a great deal of time into collecting data and very little time into thinking about how to present it. However, how you present your data often determines whether your intended audience understands your work or is even interested in it. (Teachers are all aware of this point!) The most common choice for presentations is a frequency distribution, which shows the frequency of each measure of a variable. You can add up these frequencies and create either cumulative frequency columns or grouped frequencies, depending on the question you are trying to answer.

You can also calculate percentages, which are parts of the whole. Because many nurses are familiar with them, percentages are sometimes a useful way to convey information. You can then add up the percentages and present a cumulative percentage, which is simply the percentage of observations with a value less than the maximum value of the interval.

Another way to convey information is with a visual graph, such as a bar chart for nominal data, a histogram for ordinal or continuous data, a line graph for continuous variables that change over time, or a scatterplot in which one subject's values for two variables are graphed. You need to decide which type of chart will work the best for the audience you are trying to reach. Just remember, use color, make it bigger, avoid just using lots and lots of numbers in a row, and bring coffee because most nurses are considerably sleep deprived!

CHAPTER 2 REVIEW QUESTIONS

1. A study of 30 fathers was completed in which the fathers were asked the highest level of education they had completed. Ten completed only elementary school; 10 completed elementary and high school; 7 completed elementary, high school, and college; and 3 completed elementary, high school, college, and graduate school. What was the cumulative percentage of fathers who completed only elementary school?

2. In your study of 40 people, 8 had no cold symptoms, 12 had mild cold symptoms, 9 had moderate cold symptoms, and 10 had severe cold symptoms. One patient was lost to follow-up. What percentage of patients reported cold symptoms?

3. Given the information in question 2, what percentage of patients reported no cold symptoms?

(continues)

4. Use the frequency distribution in Figure 2-12 to construct a bar chart for influenza cases in your hospital during 8 months of 2010. How would your chart look different if it were a histogram? Discuss at least one rationale for selecting either a bar chart or a histogram to present this data.

_____

_____

_____

Figure 2-12 Influenza Cases for 2010.

Month	Number of Cases
August	18
September	29
October	68
November	107
December	158
January	166
February	160
March	111

Questions 5–7: Your community begins a large-scale influenza vaccine effort, and the following year the number of cases drops (see Figure 2-13).

Figure 2-13 Influenza Cases for 2011.

Month	Number of Cases
August	19
September	27
October	31
November	34
December	48
January	59
February	51
March	45

(continues)

5. Construct a line graph showing the data from 2010 and the data from 2011. Compare the two.

6. Why didn't the numbers change significantly for August and September?

_____

7. Do you consider the vaccine effort to be successful? Why?

_____

_____

Research Application

Questions 8–13: See the data in Figure 2-14.

8. Construct a bar chart for mother's marital status.

9. What percentage of the adolescents are employed? What percentage of the adolescents are in school? Are these variables quantitative or qualitative?

_____

_____

_____

10. Identify the level of measurement of each variable.

_____

_____

_____

11. Could any of these variables have been measured as continuous quantitative variables?

_____

Figure 2-14 Demographic Characteristics of 92 Adolescents Completing a Family Planning Survey.

	n (%)
Pregnancy status	
Pregnant	78 (84.7)
Not pregnant	14 (15.2)
Age	
≤ 14 years old	2 (2.2)
15–17 years old	46 (50)
18–19 years old	43 (46.7)
Number in household[*]	
< 6 people	70 (79.5)
≥ 6 people	18 (20.5)
Student status[†]	
Not in school	46 (50.5)
In school	45 (49.4)
Mother's marital status	
Single	38 (41.3)
Married	27 (29.3)
Divorced	13 (14.1)
Other	14 (15.2)
Employment status	
Employed	25 (27.2)
Not employed	67 (72.8)

[*]Missing *n* = 4

[†]Missing *n* = 1

Source: Heavey, E., Moysich, K., Hyland, A., Druschel, C., & Sill, M. Female adolescents' perception of male partners' pregnancy desire. *Journal of Midwifery and Women's Health*, 53(4), 338–344. Copyright Elsevier (2008). Used with permission.

12. Construct a histogram for the ages of the adolescents. Describe the histogram's shape and what it tells you about this sample population. Why would a histogram be an appropriate choice for presenting this data?

(continues)

13. Is the pregnancy status of this group of adolescents typical? Why might that be?

_____

_____

14. You've been recruited by the president of FEMA to act as the head triage nurse for a large city's hurricane response team. One of your main duties is to decide which nurses will cover which facilities in the overall relief effort. Because most nursing duties will have to change during this shift in personnel, you decide to divide the group based on years of experience. Your nurse's aide carries out a brief survey of all the personnel available (100 nurses) and gives you a list of number of years of experience for each (see Figure 2-15). Find the quartiles of this distribution, and assign a role to each nurse. For example, the nurses with the least amount of experience should be assigned to the rescue team, and the ones with the most experience should be assigned to the ICU.

_____

_____

Figure 2-15 Nurses Available for the Hurricane Response Team.

Number of Years Experience	Number of Nurses	Number of Years Experience	Number of Nurses
2	15	12	3
3	10	13	3
4	9	15	3
5	8	18	3
6	8	20	2
7	9	25	2
8	6	32	1
9	5	35	1
10	5	36	1
11	5	40	1

Coordinated Hurricane Response

Rescue Team   Stadium   Hospital   ICU

Use your computer to practice these applications. The companion website for this book has a computer-based application example for this material. Check it out!

Analyze	Graphs	Utilities	Add-ons	Window	Help
Reports		▶			
Descriptive Statistics		▶	123 Frequencies...		

ANSWERS TO CHAPTER 2 REVIEW QUESTIONS

1. 33%

3. 20%

5. Answer includes line graph; beginning in October there is a substantial decrease in cases.

7. Yes, there was a substantial decrease in cases beginning in October after the vaccine was administered.

9. 27.2%, 49.4%, qualitative

11. Yes, age, number in household, years in school, years employed

13. No, all of the adolescents were waiting for pregnancy or family planning–related services.

Chapter 3

Descriptive Statistics, Probability, and Measures of Central Tendency

What does the data tell me?

OBJECTIVES

By the end of this chapter students will be able to:

- Compare and contrast descriptive statistics and inferential statistics.

- Define, distinguish between, and interpret the mean, median, mode, and standard deviation.

- Identify unimodal, bimodal, and multimodal distributions.

- Determine which measure of central tendency is appropriate in a given data set.

- Calculate and interpret a standard deviation and range for a given data set.

- Explain descriptive results from a given data set using an SPSS (Statistical Package for the Social Sciences) printout.

- Define probability and explain the range of possible probabilities.

- Compare and contrast frequency and probability distributions.

- Contrast positive and negative distribution skews and describe where the outliers are present.

KEY TERMS

Bimodal
Having two values or categories that have the highest occurrence and that are equal frequencies.

Central tendency
An indicator of the center of the data.

Frequency distribution
Lists all the possible outcomes of an experiment and tallies the number of times each outcome occurs.

Mean
The sum of the values divided by the total number of observations. It is the most commonly known measure of central tendency but requires interval or ratio data.

Median
For ordinal, interval, and ratio data, the value in the middle when you line up all the measured values in order from least to most, the 50th percentile value.

Mode
The most frequently occurring value or category in the distribution.

Multimodal
Having more than two modes.

Normal curve
A probability distribution in which the mean, median and mode are equal.

Probability distribution
Shows the probability of all the possible outcomes of the variable.

Probability
The chance that a particular outcome will occur after an event.

Range
The difference between the maximum and minimum values in a distribution.

Sampling distributions
Plots *realized* frequencies of a statistic versus the range of *possible* values that statistic can take.

Skewness
An asymmetrical distribution of the values of the variable around the mean, making one tail longer than the other.

Standard deviation
The average distance the values in a distribution are from the center.

Descriptive Statistics: Properties of Variables

Once the variables of interest in a study have been defined, nurses and statisticians usually look at a set of so-called descriptive statistics that allow them to get to know more about each variable. A variable can be described in two main ways:

- In terms of its central value or tendency.
- In terms of how far away from the variable's center the observations are spread.

We'll start by defining central tendency.

Measures of Central Tendency

Central tendency is an indicator of the center of the data. Defining the central tendency of a distribution more specifically, however, is not easy because the answer depends on the analysis technique used—which in turn depends on the level of measurement of the data. Let's start by remembering the levels of measurement.

First, *nominal variables* describe categorical differences, such as gender. The only measure of central tendency for nominal data is the **mode**, which is the most frequently occurring measure in the data. For example, if your sample includes 15 men and 5 women, the mode is the 15 men. If a ZIP code sample includes 7 people living in 14617, 7 people living in 14619, and 6 living in 14621. The two values (14617 and 14619) have the highest occurrence and are equal; so the sample has two modes and is called bimodal. Large samples may even be **multimodal**, that is, have more than two modes.

Data that is rank ordered (ordinal, interval, or ratio) has a second measure of central tendency: a **median**. If you line up all the measured values in order from least to most, the value in the middle of the list is the median. For example, suppose a set of students have the following scores on the last nursing exam: 66, 74, 83, 83, 88, 94, 96, 97, 99. The median score is 88, the one right in the middle. Or suppose that the first person who takes the exam forgets to hand it in so that the number of exams is even: 74, 83, 83, 88, 94, 96, 97, 99. Then the median is actually the average of the fourth and fifth values: (88 + 94) ÷ 2, or 91%.

The mode in this data is 83. You can see that the measures of central tendency do not always produce the same results. This is the main reason why defining central tendency is difficult.

Perhaps the most commonly known measure of central tendency is the **mean**, which is the sum of the values divided by the total number of observations. For example, if you add up all the original test scores and divide by the total number who took the test, you find that the mean of the original test scores is 86.67: (66 + 74 + 83 + 83 + 88 + 94 + 96 + 97 + 99) ÷ 9. Again, the mean is not the same as the median or the mode. Each is a different measure of central tendency. They may even be the same number (as in a normal distribution, which we talk about later), but they do not have to be and they all have different definitions. The mean can be calculated only if the available data is at the interval or ratio level. You cannot calculate a mean on ordinal or nominal data. Think about it: What is the "average" gender? That doesn't make sense. Nominal or ordinal data does not lend itself to the calculation of averages. However, even with interval- or ratio-level data, you may decide to use the median instead of the mean for your measure of central tendency. This is frequently considered the better option.

Why is the median considered a better statistic to use than the mean? Students in any course should be *very* interested in the answer. Let's say the following scores are recorded on a final exam:

32, 35, 38, 40, 41, 41, 42, 43, 44,
45, 46, 47, 48, 99, 100, 100

Clearly, the class, overall, did not do very well on this exam. In fact, of the 16 people who took the exam, only 3 passed, scoring significantly higher than the rest of the class. These three scores are outliers (observations that are significantly different from the rest of the sample) and may distort the mean while leaving the median relatively unaltered. Let's take a look.

- The mean of the data is 50.
- The median of the data is 43.5.

You can see that the 43.5 is a much better estimate of the central tendency, and in fact the mean is so high only because of the three top scores, which are very different from the rest of the data. If you scored a 48 on this test, you did fairly well in comparison to your classmates, scoring higher than 75% of them. However, what if your professor decided to look just at the mean? She might tell you that you didn't even beat the average grade for the class, even though only three people actually outscored you!

Range and Sample Standard Deviation

Variables can vary from their center or central tendency, and the variation can be explained by two terms.

- First, the **range** is the difference between the maximum value and minimum value of a variable. For example, in a sample there might be five subjects ages 10, 14, 20, 55, and 95. The age range of the sample is 85 years (95 years minus 10 years) or it can also be reported as 10 to 95 years.
- The **standard deviation** is the average distance of the values from the variable's mean. When the standard deviation is large, the spread among the values in the data set is large. When the deviation is small, most of the scores are very close to the average score.

You may find that, although the average heart rate is the same on a postpartum unit as on a cardiac intensive care unit, the ranges and standard deviations in the heart rates are substantially different (see Figure 3-1).

Standard deviation is harder to calculate than range, but not that hard. Suppose you collect heart rates for the patients who are day one post-delivery on your postpartum unit and find that the mean heart rate is $(45 + 60 + 75 + 90) \div 4 = 67.5$ (see Figure 3-2). The formula for the standard deviation (*SD*) is shown in Figure 3-3.

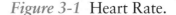

Figure 3-1 Heart Rate.

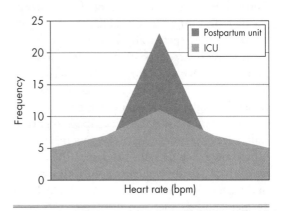

In a less "mathematical" version, it might look like this:

$$SD = \sqrt{\frac{(\text{first value} - \text{mean})^2 + (\text{second value} - \text{mean})^2 + ... + (n\text{th} - \text{mean})^2}{\text{number of values} - 1}}$$

In our example, then, the standard deviation is the square root of:

$$\frac{(45 - 67.5)^2 + (60 - 67.5)^2 + (75 - 67.5)^2 + (90 - 67.5)^2}{4 - 1}$$

This equals:

$$\frac{(-22.5)(-22.5) + (-7.5)(-7.5) + (7.5)(7.5) + (22.5)(22.5)}{3}$$

Or:

$$\frac{506.25 + 56.25 + 56.25 + 506.25}{3}$$

This comes down to what is actually called the sample variance:

$$\frac{1125}{3} = 375$$

Then you need to take the square root of 375: 19.36. So the standard deviation in the postpartum sample is 19.36.

Figure 3-2 Frequency Table for Heart Rates Day 1 Postpartum.

Heart Rate	Frequency
45	1
60	1
75	1
90	1

Figure 3-3 Calculating the Sample Standard Deviation.

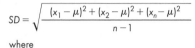

$$SD = \sqrt{\frac{(x_1 - \mu)^2 + (x_2 - \mu)^2 + (x_n - \mu)^2}{n - 1}}$$

where
x = values in the distribution
μ = mean

FROM THE STATISTICIAN · BRENDAN HEAVEY

Why Is There an n − 1 in the Denominator of Sample Variance?

Wouldn't it be a whole lot easier to remember sample variance if the denominator didn't contain an $n - 1$? The answer is yes, remembering the formula would be a heck of a lot easier if we could just scrap the $n - 1$ and throw an n into the denominator. In fact, as the sample size of our data set increases, the $n - 1$ becomes more and more negligible. However, in small samples we can see that the sample mean is a heck of a lot closer to each sample value than the population mean.

Think about it: Although the sample mean is a decent descriptor of the middle of our sample, the population mean doesn't even have to be within the range of our sample! Let's think about an example. If you were interested in estimating the average heart rate of a human being in normal sinus rhythm you might sample from 10 different healthy volunteers. Each volunteer would have small differences in their own heart rate depending on what time of day you took their pulse, how much they had been moving in the moments leading up to your measurement, their BMI, and so on. Let's say you choose to test each person's heart rate five different times, and took an average of those measurements to report on, your results might look like this:

	Person 1	Person 2	Person 3	Person 4	Person 5
	65	65	51	69	79
	62	67	58	72	72
	60	58	55	73	75
	58	62	53	70	78
	61	63	59	76	77
Sample Means	Avg = 61.2	Avg = 63	Avg = 55.2	Avg = 72	Avg = 76.2
Population Mean	Overall Average = 65.52				

(continues)

FROM THE STATISTICIAN BRENDAN HEAVEY

Take a look at how the individual pulse rates vary around their individual sample means. Notice that the overall mean is generally further away from the data points than the sample mean is. In fact, the population mean is not even in the range of Person 5's recorded values. Let's calculate the numerator of #5's variance using the sample mean. We get:

$$(79 - 76.2)^2 + (72 - 76.2)^2 + (75 - 76.2)^2 + (78 - 76.2)^2 + (77 - 76.2)^2 = 30.8$$

Now, let's do the same thing but substitute the population mean. We get:

$$(79 - 65.52)^2 + (72 - 65.52)^2 + (75 - 65.52)^2 + (78 - 65.52)^2 + (77 - 65.52)^2 = 601.112$$

Clearly, Person 5 contributes a lot more to the variance component of the population than he does to the sample. In general, there is a lot less variance around the sample mean than the population mean, so sample variance tends to underestimate the population variance. You can make up for this difference, or what the statisticians call bias, by putting an $n - 1$ in the denominator of the sample variance calculation.

Okay, now I know some of you are starting to wonder, "Why am I in this class again?" Don't get too frustrated by the equations. (If, on the other hand, you are just dying to know more about variance, please read the "From the Statistician" feature, which delves further into this topic!) The essential concept to understand is why the standard deviation is important. (*It tells you the average distance the values in your distribution fall from the mean.*)

Moving Forward: Inferential Statistics

Once researchers are done describing the variables they are interested in, they usually like to make inferences about populations based on the measurements they have taken in their samples. This practice, called inferential statistics, involves associating probabilities with each variable studied. **Probability** is the chance that a particular outcome will occur. For example, let's say a class of 100 nursing students has 25 men and 75 women, and we want to know the prob-

ability that a randomly chosen student from this class will be female. The answer is 75/100, or 0.75, or 75%. Probabilities are important because, no matter how careful and precise researchers are, there is always some level of uncertainty. Even if the researchers believe the class is composed entirely of men, the researchers cannot say the probability is 1.0, or 100%, that a randomly chosen student will be male; they can only say that the probability approaches 100%. (Did anyone see the Disney movie *Mulan*? To make a long story short a young Chinese woman joins the imperial army disguised as a man. If one were to randomly select an infantry soldier from this "all male" group, the probability that you would select a man approaches 100% but there is always room for some error such as if one were to randomly select Mulan in disguise! But I digress. . .) Conversely, the researchers cannot say that the probability of randomly selecting a female from what they believe is an all-male class is 0.0, or 0%. They can only say the probability approaches 0. Probability theory is a science in and of itself; so here we'll cover it in a nutshell in the next "From the Statistician."

FROM THE STATISTICIAN   BRENDAN HEAVEY

Probability and the Normal Distribution

Probability is a difficult concept to fully grasp. In fact, it has so many different facets that at times statisticians have a difficult time adequately defining it. The good news is that, at this point, you don't need an extremely in-depth understanding of it. In fact, for the purposes of this class, think of probability as long-run relative frequency. You know what relative frequency means (see "From the Statistician" in Chapter 2), but what does "long-run" mean? That's an important question, and it doesn't have a very good answer. Let's look at an example to try to explain this concept.

We're going to revisit the age-old experiment of rolling dice. Figure 3-4 shows the results of rolling a single die 10 times and counting how many times the die shows a 3 on its face. The cumulative and relative frequencies associated with each roll are tabulated in the last two columns, just as we did in Chapter 2. This time, we're going to focus on that final column, the relative frequency. The relative frequency is the total number of times you roll a particular value (in this case, 3) out of the total number of rolls.

If you look at the relative frequency column closely, you will notice that it starts out low and then, as soon as we roll a 3, the relative frequency jumps up to 0.5. In fact, if we continued this experiment for a long time, the jumping would continue forever—each time you roll another 3 and increase the numerator. However, each jump would be smaller than the last (because each roll also increases the denominator).

Just for fun, we did this very thing and plotted the relative frequency over 1000 rolls in Figure 3-5. Notice that, after a while, the relative frequency of rolling a 3 settles down to around 0.16, or 1/6. In the beginning, the relative frequency jumps up and down, but after about 100 rolls, we can clearly see the trend settling. We would fully expect this going forward because the die has six sides, and if we rolled the die a million times, we would expect somewhere around 1/6 of them to turn up a 3. In this experiment, because we can see the main pattern developed after 100 rolls, we would define "long run" as 100 rolls, but keep in mind that the definition can change between experiments.

Figure 3-4 Frequency Table for Rolling a 3 When Rolling a 6-sided Die.

Roll	Result	Cumulative Frequency of 3	Relative Frequency of 3
1	1	0	0
2	3	1	½ = 0.5
3	2	1	⅓ = 0.33
4	5	1	¼ = 0.25
5	6	1	⅕ = 0.2
6	2	1	⅙ = 0.16
7	3	2	2/7 = 0.29
8	4	2	2/8 = 0.25
9	4	2	2/9 = 0.22
10	6	2	2/10 = 0.2

Figure 3-5 Graph of the Relative Frequency of Rolling a 3.

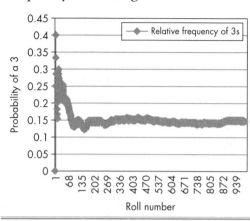

Frequency Distributions Versus Probability Distributions

From Chapter 2, you will remember that a **frequency distribution** simply lists all the possible outcomes of an experiment and tallies the number of times each outcome occurs. These tallies are then graphed to make them easier to visualize and comprehend. A **probability distribution** graphs the probability of all the possible outcomes of the variable instead of their frequency. Although they both look a lot alike, they represent two very distinct concepts.

Let's look more in depth at the difference between a frequency distribution and a probability distribution. The frequency distribution for the experiment of rolling a die 1000 times is shown in Figure 3-6 and compared against the probability distribution of rolling a die indefinitely. As you can see, the frequency distribution has notches and changes depending on what a sample looks like. The probability distribution is uniform and never changes. The relationship between relative frequency and probability closely resembles the relationship between a

sample and a population. The difference boils down to a basic difference between the short run (100 tosses of the die) and the long run (1000, 10,000, 100,000 tosses?), and defining the long run is slightly subjective.

That's great, you might say, "But we're nurses! We're never going to need to roll dice and come up with associated probabilities unless we meet a poor statistician sitting at a bar all alone somewhere!" Nevertheless, as it turns out, rolling a die is just a very straightforward example of an experiment. Let's consider a couple of basic experiments and see how they might relate to your life and profession. For instance, we can now easily answer the following:

- What is the long-run relative frequency (or probability) of a fair coin turning up heads?
- What is the long-run relative frequency (or probability) of a fair die rolling a 6?

Now, let's look at answering some questions we're more interested in:

- What is the probability that I will die of cardiovascular disease?
- What is the probability that one of my patients will be discharged before I come back to the hospital to work my next shift?
- What is the probability that a new drug will kill a cancerous tumor in my patient's liver without killing my patient?

Answering these questions with any degree of accuracy requires a lot of study, a lot of repeated samples, and determining probability—as you just did!

The Normal Distribution

Many variables of interest to us have a probability distribution that closely resembles a very famous distribution: the **normal distribution**, a probability distribution in which the mean, median, and mode are equal (see Figure 3-7). In fact, one

Figure 3-6 Frequency Versus Probability Distribution.

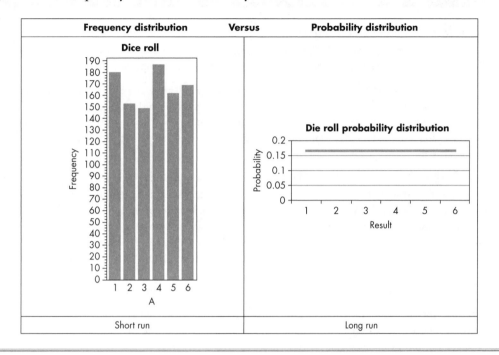

of the most common assumptions in basic research is that the variables have probability distributions that can be estimated with the normal distribution. The normal distribution is what all of us have heard of as the "bell curve." Yes, this is how grades are "curved" when no one does well on a test. Many people believe that, given a well constructed exam administered to a large enough sample, we should expect a grade distribution that can be estimated with the normal distribution.

Because in the normal distribution the mean, median, and mode are the same, you know two things about a variable that is normally distributed (see Figure 3-7):

- 68% of its values fall within one standard deviation of the mean.
- 95% of its values fall within two standard deviations of the mean.

Figure 3-7 Normal Distribution.

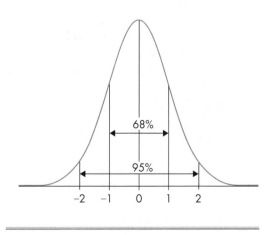

FROM THE STATISTICIAN   BRENDAN HEAVEY

What Is a Normal Distribution?

For most researchers, the normal distribution is the most important distribution in all of statistics. Two very important facts about the normal distribution make it so important:

1. If you take the mean from lots and lots of samples of a population, the distribution of the sample means (the sampling distribution of the mean) becomes normal in the long run. Sampling distributions plot *actual* frequencies of a statistic versus the range of *possible* values that statistic can take.
2. As you add more and more random variables together, their overall distribution approaches the normal distribution.

In Figure 3-8, check out how the plot of the normal distribution looks as you adjust its mean. As the mean (μ) of the distribution increases in these graphs, the curve shifts to the right; as it decreases, the curve shifts to the left. This shift is why we call the mean a location parameter.

In Figure 3-9, see what happens when we change the variance. If we were to change only the variance (σ) in our formula, we would see a change in scale. As we decrease the variance, the graph gets taller and skinnier, and as we increase it, the graph gets shorter and fatter. That is why variance is called a scale variable.

Here are some more important things we know about the normal distribution:

- 68% of the area under the curve falls within 1 standard deviation of the mean.
- 95% of the area under the curve falls within 2 standard deviations of the mean.
- Increasing the mean makes the curve shift to the right.
- Decreasing the mean makes the curve shift to the left.
- Decreasing the variance makes the graph look taller and skinnier.
- Increasing the variance makes it look short and fat.

An important thing we can do with any normal variable is transform its distribution into a *standard* normal distribution. This forces all the area under the curve to fall under the normal curve with a mean of 0 and a standard deviation of 1. We do this with the transformation formula shown in Figure 3-10. If Y is a normally distributed variable, this equation will produce Z, which is a standard normal variable. Standard normal variables are great because we know a lot about their probabilities. For instance, 5% of the probability is found beyond $Z = 1.96$.

Skewed Distributions

Of course, not all samples are normally distributed. For example, some samples are **skewed**; they have an asymmetrical distribution of the values of the variable around the mean so that one tail is longer than the other. See Figure 3-11. Skewing is usually due to a significant number of outliers. When the outliers are on the right, the skew is positive; if most of the outliers are on the left, the skew is negative. In skewed distributions, the mean, median, and mode are not equal. Remember the test where you got a 48 but only three people scored higher? That is an example of a positive skew produced by outliers.

Figure 3-8 Normal Distribution: Changing the Mean.

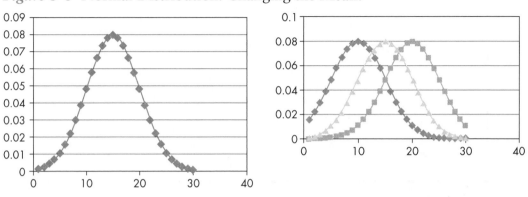

Summary

Congratulate yourself for making it through Chapter 3! Let's restate some main points from this very detailed chapter.

When you have nominal-level data, the only measure of central tendency you can use is the mode. The mode is the most frequently occurring measure in a distribution. A bimodal distribution has two values with the highest number of frequencies an equal number of times; this gives you two modes. Taking that one step

further, a multimodal distribution has more than two modes.

The median can be used with ordinal, interval, or ratio data and is found by lining up the measured values in order from least to greatest and locating the value in the middle. For interval- or ratio-level data, you can also calculate a mean or average. The mean is the most commonly known measure of central tendency and is found by taking the sum of the values divided by the total number of observations.

With regard to the dispersion of your data, two terms are important: (1) the range, or the difference between the maximum and minimum values in the distribution, and (2) the standard deviation, or the average distance of the values in a distribution from the center.

Everyone's favorite concept in statistics is the symmetrical normal distribution, often

Figure 3-9 Normal Distribution: Changing the Variance.

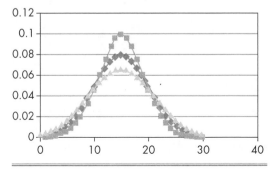

Figure 3-10 Formula for Creating a Standard Normal Variable.

$$Z = \frac{Y - \mu}{\sigma} \sim N(0,\ 1)$$

Figure 3-11 Skewed Distributions.

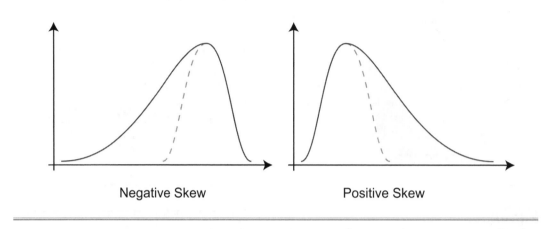

represented by the bell curve. If your data fits into this type of distribution, it simplifies your analysis immensely.

Some samples are skewed; that is, they have an asymmetrical distribution of the values of the variable around the mean so that one tail is larger than the other. If you have this type of sample distribution, you need to make adjustments before applying some of the simpler analysis techniques.

If you understand these main concepts, you are on the right track and are ready to go on to the next chapter—or take a long nap. Personally, I would probably vote for the nap first anyhow!

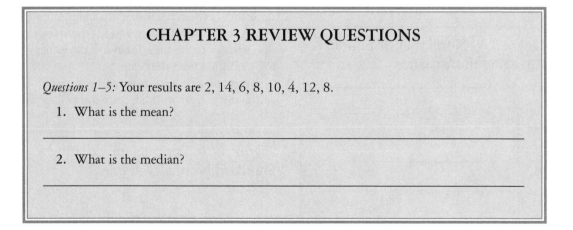

CHAPTER 3 REVIEW QUESTIONS

Questions 1–5: Your results are 2, 14, 6, 8, 10, 4, 12, 8.

1. What is the mean?

2. What is the median?

3. What is the mode?

_____

4. Calculate the standard deviation.

_____

5. If the sample is normally distributed, 68% of the responses are within what range?

_____

6. If a study reports that you have a normally distributed sample with a mean age of 17.3 years, what is the median?

_____

Questions 7–12: A study polls 40 new mothers who attempt to nurse their infants from birth to six weeks. Twenty-seven mothers report nursing with minimal pain and frustration, 10 mothers report nursing with moderate pain and frustration, and 3 mothers report discontinuing nursing due to high levels of pain and frustration.

7. What is the mode for nursing pain and frustration?

_____

8. What is the median for nursing pain and frustration?

_____

9. What percentage of mothers continued to nurse for the full six weeks with minimal pain and frustration?

_____

10. What percentage of mothers reported less than or equal to moderate pain and frustration?

_____

11. What level of measurement is the nursing pain and frustration?

_____

12. How could you increase the level of measurement?

_____

(continues)

Questions 13–18: You read a study involving a new screen for rheumatoid arthritis, and the report indicates that those with the disease had the antibody levels shown in Figure 3-12.

Figure 3-12 Frequency Table for Rheumatoid Arthritis Screen.

Antibody Level	Frequency	Cumulative Frequency
20	3	————
30	5	————
43	3	————
48	7	————

13. Complete the cumulative frequency column.

14. How many subjects had their antibody levels reported?

_____

15. What antibody level was the mode?

_____

16. What antibody level was the median?

_____

17. What antibody level was the mean?

_____

18. Is this sample normally distributed?

_____

Questions 19–21: Final exam grades are normally distributed with a mean of 81. The standard deviation is 3.

19. What range includes 68% of the sample?

_____

20. What range includes 95% of the sample?

_____

21. What is the median grade?

_____

_____

Questions 22–26: A researcher is measuring how many times a minute a person coughs when exposed to cigarette smoke. The results from the study are normally distributed, and they include a mean of 4 and a standard deviation of 2.

22. What level of measurement is this?

_____

23. What is an appropriate measure of central tendency?

_____

24. Where do 68% of the sample responses fall?

_____

25. If instead the results show a mean of 4 and a standard deviation of 1 but remain normally distributed, what would this change do to the curve?

_____

26. The follow-up cohort study reports a mean of 5 and a standard deviation of 1. What would this change do to the curve?

_____

_____

Questions 27–31: A sample of orthopedic patients on your unit includes:
    Two patients on intravenous anticoagulants.
    Four patients on oral anticoagulants.
    Two patients on subcutaneous anticoagulants.

27. Based on this sample, calculate the probability that orthopedic patients are given IV anticoagulants?

_____

28. Calculate the probability that orthopedic patients are given oral anticoagulants?

_____

29. Calculate the probability that orthopedic patients are given subcutaneous anticoagulants?

_____

(continues)

30. Based on this sample, what is the probability that an orthopedic patient will be given some form of anticoagulant?

31. Hip replacement patients have the same probability of being on oral anticoagulants as the orthopedic patients in your previous study, and you have four in your daily assignment. Calculate the number of the patients with hip replacements who you would anticipate would need oral anticoagulants.

Use your computer to practice these applications. The companion website for this book has a computer-based application example for this material. Check it out!

ANSWERS TO CHAPTER 3 REVIEW QUESTIONS

1. 8

3. 8

5. Between 4 and 12

7. Minimal

9. 67.5%

11. Ordinal

13. 3, 8, 11, 18

15. Mode $= 48$

17. Mean $= 37.5$

19. 78–84

21. 81

23. Any

25. Make it taller and skinnier

27. $\frac{2}{8} = \frac{1}{4} = 25\%$

29. $\frac{2}{8} = \frac{1}{4} = 25\%$

31. 2

Evaluating Your Measurement Tool

Is your instrument good, bad, or ugly?

OBJECTIVES

By the end of the chapter students will be able to:

- Discuss factors which impact the feasibility of a study.

- Define validity and why it is essential in research.

- Identify various methods for establishing validity, and give an example of each.

- Define reliability and relate why it is important in research.

- Describe the main components of reliability.

- Detect when inter-rater reliability needs to be assessed and develop a plan for doing so.

- Formulate a 2 × 2 table, and calculate the sensitivity and specificity of a screening test from a given data set.

- Distinguish between sensitivity and specificity, and identify when each is important.

- Calculate the positive and negative predictive value of a screening test.

- Calculate the prevalence of an illness and describe how the positive and negative predictive values of the screening test are affected by the prevalence of the illness among the test population.

- Critique a screening test utilizing a given data set.

- Prepare an argument for why or why not a particular screen should be utilized based on current research.

KEY TERMS

Content validity
When the instrument used is designed to accurately measure the concepts under study.

Convergent validity
When your results are similar to the results obtained with another previously validated test that measures the same thing.

Divergent validity
When the measurement of the opposite variable of a previously validated measurement yields the opposite result.

Efficiency
Measures the probability of agreement between the screening test and the actual clinical diagnosis.

Equivalence
How well multiple forms or multiple users of an instrument produce the same results.

Feasible
Possible from a practical standpoint.

Homogeneity
The extent to which items on a multi-item instrument are consistent with one another.

Inter-rater reliability
When you compare the measurements obtained by two different data collectors to make sure they are similar.

Internal consistency reliability
Homogeneity of the measurement instrument.

Negative predictive value
If the subject tests negative for a disease the probability that the subject really doesn't have the disease.

Positive predictive value (PPV)
If a subject tests positive for a disease, the probability that the subject actually has the disease and that the result isn't a false positive.

Predictive validity
When the instrument used accurately suggests future outcomes or behaviors.

Prevalence
The amount of illness present in the population divided by the total population.

Reliability
The consistency or repeatability of the measurement.

Sensitivity
If the patient has the disease, the probability of a positive test result for the disease (the probability of a true positive).

Specificity
The probability that a well subject will have a negative screen (no disease) (the probability of a true negative).

Stability
The consistent or enduring quality of the measure.

Valid
Accurate.

Feasibility

Before selecting any type of research instrument you should always assess the **feasibility** or practicality of the tool. If, for example, you want to use computer assisted interviewing techniques to survey adolescents about sexual behavior but your grant is for $1,000, and each device is $1,200 it is probably not a practical plan. A study that involves asking patients with dementia to complete a 24 hour recall of food consumption also lacks feasibility. A wise nurse will consider the practical aspects of the study's measurement tool such as the cost, time, training and the limitations of your study sample (physical, cultural, educational, psychosocial, etc.) before beginning the analysis of the validity and reliability of the instruments themselves.

Validity

After you determine that your instrument is feasible for use in your study you can then proceed to assess the validity and reliability of your tool. The information you gather is helpful only if your measurement and collection methods are accurate, or **valid**. You can ensure that an instrument has validity in several ways:

- *Determine relevant variables from a thorough literature search:* When you began your research, you did a literature search to determine what information, if any, was already available about the relationship between family visits and the length of recovery time needed after a hip replacement.
- *Include the variables in a measurement instrument:* In your literature search, you identified some of the major variables to consider in your study, such as the support level of family members, the age of the patient,

whether the patient lives alone, whether this was the patient's first surgery, and other factors.
- *Have your instrument reviewed by experts for feedback:* When you designed the survey for your study, you included these variables and then had your nurse manager, two nursing researchers, and your fellowship advisor (all experts) review your survey.

These steps are all part of ensuring **content validity**.

You can also show validity in your survey by comparing your results with those of a previously validated survey that measures the same thing. This type of comparison is called **convergent validity**. For example, if you find a correlation of 0.4 or higher, that finding strengthens the validity of both instruments, yours and the previous one (Grove, 2007). (Note: We discuss correlation coefficients in Chapter 11.) In turn, if your survey is later found to be able to predict the length of stay for those admitted in the future, that finding will strengthen the validity of your instrument and your study would have **predictive validity** as well.

Some instruments are considered valid because they measure the opposite variable of a previously validated measurement and find the opposite result. For instance, suppose a group of people with elevated serum cholesterol levels, also scored low on a survey you designed to measure intake of fruits and vegetables. This result is an example of **divergent validity** in your instrument. The group with high cholesterol also had a poor diet. If the negative correlation is greater than or equal to -0.4, the divergent validity of both measures is strengthened (Grove, 2007).

Another way to show validity with opposite results is if your instrument detects a difference in groups already known to have a difference.

This is also referred to as construct validity testing using known groups. For example, you are testing a new instrument to examine labor outcomes in women who have already had a baby versus those experiencing their first labor. The instrument measures length of labor, which has already been shown to be shorter for women who have had a baby. You find that those who have had a baby have a length of labor that is on average two hours shorter than those who have not. This finding supports the validity of your new measurement tool because it detected a difference that was known to exist.

Reliability

Reliability means that your measurement tool is consistent or repeatable. When you measure your variable of interest, do you get the same results every time? Reliability is different from accuracy or validity. Suppose, for example, that you are measuring the weight of the study participants, but your scale is not calibrated correctly; it's off by 20 pounds. You get the same measure every time the patient steps on the scale; that is, the measurement is repeatable and reliable. However, in this case it is not accurate or valid. A measure can be reliable and not valid, but it can't be valid and not reliable. Think of it this way; For an instrument to be accurate (valid), it must be accurate and reliable.

Three main factors relate to reliability: stability, homogeneity and equivalence.

Stability is the consistent or enduring quality of the measure. A stable measure should:

- Not change over time.
- And, when administered repeatedly, it should have a high correlation coefficient. (The correlation coefficient measures how closely one measurement is related to a second measurement. For example, if you mea-

sure the temperature of a healthy individual six times in an hour, the readings should be approximately the same and have a high correlation coefficient. Of course, that patient may be really sick of having you around, but I am sure your excitement at discovering that you have a stable measure will make it all worthwhile! Again, see Chapter 11.)

You need to evaluate the stability of your measurement instrument at the beginning of the study and throughout it. For example, if your thermometer breaks, the instrument that was once stable is no longer available. Your ongoing results are no longer reliable, and you need to have a protocol to figure out quickly how to reestablish stability.

The second quality of a reliable measure, **homogeneity**, is the extent to which items on a multi-item instrument are consistent with each other. For example, your survey may ask several questions designed to measure the level of family support. The questions may be repeated but worded differently to see whether the individuals completing the survey respond in the same way. One question may ask, "What level of family support do you feel on most days?" And the choices may be high, medium, and low. Later in the survey you may ask the individual to indicate on a scale of one to ten how supported they feel by their family on an average day. If the instrument has homogeneity, those who answered that they had, say, a medium level of family support on most days should also be somewhere around the middle of the one-to-ten scale. If so, then your instrument is said to have **internal consistency reliability**.

Internal consistency reliability is useful for instruments that measure a single concept, such as family support, and is frequently assessed using Cronbach's alpha. Cronbach's alpha ranges from 0 (no reliability in the instrument scale) to

1 (perfect reliability in the instrument scale) so the higher value indicates better internal consistency reliability. You may hear more about this test in future statistics or research classes, but right now you just need to know that it can be used to establish homogeneity or internal consistency reliability (Nieswiadomy, 2008).

The third factor relating to reliability is **equivalence**. Equivalence is how well multiple forms of an instrument or multiple users of an instrument produce/obtain the same results. Measurement variation is a reflection of more than the reliability of the tool itself; it may also reflect the variability of different forms of the tool or variability due to different researchers administering the same tool. For example, if you want to observe the color of scrubs worn by 60 nurses at lunchtime on a particular day, you might need help in gathering that much data in such a short period of time. You might ask two research assistants to observe the nurses. When you have more than one individual collecting data, you should determine the **inter-rater reliability**. One way to do this is to have all three individuals who are collecting data observe the first five nurses together and then classify the data individually. For example:

- You say the first five nurses are wearing: blue, green, green, orange, and pink scrubs.
- The second research assistant reports that the first five nurses are wearing: teal, lime, lime, tangerine, and rose scrubs.
- The third reports that the first five nurses are wearing: blue, green, green, orange, and pink scrubs.

In this example, the inter-rater reliability between you and the third data collector is 100%, whereas it is 0% between you and the second collector. You have clearly identified a problem with the instrument's inter-rater reliability.

One way to increase reliability is to create color categories for data collection: blue, green, orange, yellow, and other. In this case:

- You report the first five nurses are wearing blue, green, green, orange, and other.
- The second data collector reports the nurses are wearing blue, green, green, other, and other.
- The third data collector matches your selections again.

Clearly you have improved the inter-rater reliability, but some variability is left due to the collectors' differences in interpretation of colors. With this information, you may decide that the help of second data collector isn't worth the loss in inter-rater reliability. You might run the study with only two data collectors, or you may decide to sit down, define specific colors with the second data collector, and then reexamine the inter-rater reliability. In all such cases, you must consider this concern whenever the study requires more than one data collector.

The readability of an instrument can also affect both the validity and reliability of the tool. If your study participants cannot understand the words in your survey tool, there is a very good chance they will not complete it accurately or consistently and that would ruin all your hard work. A good researcher assesses the readability of her instrument before or during the pilot stage of her study.

One last point to remember is that the validity and reliability of an instrument are not inherent attributes of the instrument but are characteristics of the use of the instrument with a particular group of respondents at a particular time. For example, an instrument that has been shown to be valid and reliable when used with an urban elderly population may not be valid and reliable when used with a rural adolescent population. For this reason, the validity and reliability of an instrument should be reassessed whenever that instrument is used in a new situation.

Screening Tests

Different but related terms are utilized when a screening test is selected. The accuracy of a screening test is determined by its ability to identify subjects who have the disease and subjects who do not. However, accuracy does not mean that all subjects who have a positive screen have the disease and that all subjects who have a negative screen do not.

The four possible outcomes from any screening test are best illustrated in a standard 2×2 table, also called a contingency table (see Figure 4-1).

- If a subject actually has the disease and the screen is positive, the result is a true positive and belongs in the first box (A).
- If the subject does not have the disease and the screen is positive, it is a false positive and belongs in the second box (B).
- If the subject has the disease and tests negative, it is a false negative result and belongs in the third box (C).
- If the subject does not have the disease and the screen is negative, it is a true negative and belongs in the fourth box (D).

Sensitivity

When evaluating a screening test, one of the things nurses like to know is, if the patient has the disease, what is the probability that he or she will test positive for the disease. This is known as the **sensitivity** of the test and can be calculated by the equation in Figure 4-2. Intuitively, this equation should make sense. Take the number of subjects who are sick and test positive, and divide this number by the total number of subjects who are ill. It's a matter of percentages: the number who are really sick and who test positive divided by the total number of people who really are sick. If a screen is sensitive, it is very good at identifying people who are actually sick, and it has a low percentage of false negatives. Sensitivity is particularly important when a disease is fatal or contagious or when early treatment helps.

Specificity

Another piece of information that helps evaluate a screening tool is the **specificity**, or the probability that a well subject will have a negative screen (no disease). Using the same 2×2 table, **specificity** can be calculated with the equation in Figure 4-3. Again, this equation takes the number of people who are not ill and who have a negative screening test and divides this number by the total number of people who are not ill.

Figure 4-1 2×2 Table.

	Disease Present	Disease Not Present
Test positive	True positive (A)	False positive (B)
Test negative	False negative (C)	True negative (D)

Figure 4-2 Formula to Calculate the Sensitivity of a Screen.

$$\text{Sensitivity} = \frac{A \text{ (True positives)}}{A + C \text{ (All who have the disease)}}$$

Figure 4-3 Formula to Calculate the Specificity of a Screen.

$$\text{Specificity} = \frac{\text{True negatives (D)}}{\text{All those who do not have the disease (B + D)}}$$

When a screen is highly specific, it is very good at identifying subjects who are not ill and has a low percentage of false positives.

Sensitivity and specificity tend to work in a converse balance with each other, and sometimes a loss in one is traded for an improvement in another. For example, suppose you are a nurse working on an infectious disease outbreak in a mobile military unit overseas. Your ability to find these patients again is very limited so you want to be as certain as possible that those you screen negative and leave the mobile facility are not really carrying the disease for which you are screening. Because of this you select a highly specific test which is very good at identifying those who do not have the disease for which you are screening. It rarely says a healthy person is sick. When a highly specific test is negative you know the chances are very good that the person is actually healthy and can leave the facility without a concern that they could spread the disease for which you are screening. You can then hold or contain those who do test positive for further testing and evaluation.

FROM THE STATISTICIAN   BRENDAN HEAVEY

Sensitivity and Specificity

Let's review some concepts in this chapter in the context of testing a large group of individuals for tuberculosis. For instance, when you entered nursing school, you were probably subjected to tests to determine whether you carried tuberculosis. The first step in the testing process is a PPD, which shows whether a person has antibodies to the bacterium that causes tuberculosis. A person who responds to this test may be asked to undergo any number of tests, including:

- A chest x-ray
- Biopsy
- Urine culture
- Cerebrospinal fluid sample
- CT scan
- MRI scan

(continues)

FROM THE STATISTICIAN BRENDAN HEAVEY

Each of these tests has a number of different characteristics. They can all be used in the diagnosis of tuberculosis infection, but which test is best? This question turns out to be very challenging, and the answer depends on the definition of "best." Further, each person's definition of best can be different and can change depending on that individual's perception of reality! For instance, each test costs a different amount to administer; so is the cheapest test the best? (If you thought you had tuberculosis, cost would probably not be your criterion for best.) Each test also ranges in its degree of invasiveness. Would you want to be subjected to a cerebrospinal fluid sample (think *ouch*—very painful) if you didn't think you had the disease and just wanted to get into nursing school!

Each of these tests has a different sensitivity and specificity. A very important trait of each test that you should be interested to know is how often a person **with** tuberculosis is actually diagnosed correctly. A second trait of interest is how often a person **without** tuberculosis is correctly diagnosed. In general, a high sensitivity/lower specificity test is administered first to determine a large set of people who *may* have the disease. Sensitive tests are very good at identifying those who have a disease. Then additional costs and tests are incurred to increase specificity, or eliminate people who are actually healthy (and were false positives) before diagnosis and treatment begins.

This approach is like using a microscope. The first step is to use a low-resolution lens to find the area of a slide that you're interested in. Then you increase the resolution to look more closely at the object of interest. A test with high sensitivity/low specificity is like a low-resolution lens to identify those who may have the disease. As you increase specificity, you narrow down the population of interest and eliminate those who were falsely testing positive. An example of this practice is included in Doering et al. (2007).

Positive Predictive Value of a Screen

Another important concept to understand about any screening test is **positive predictive value (PPV)**. PPV tells you what the probability is that a subject actually has the disease given a positive test result—that is, the probability of a true positive. Look back at the 2 × 2 table in Figure 4-3. You can calculate the PPV with the equation in Figure 4-4.

Unfortunately, many students find this concept confusing because it depends not just on the sensitivity and specificity of the test, but also on the prevalence of the illness in the population you are screening. **Prevalence** is the amount of illness (the number of cases) present in the population divided by the total population. If you look back at the 2 × 2 table you can determine the prevalence quite easily. It is just the number of people who have the disease divided by the total population (see Figure 4-5).

Figure 4-4 Formula to Calculate the Positive Predictive Value of a Screen.

$$PPV = \frac{\text{True positives (A)}}{\text{Total number who tested positive (A + B)}}$$

Figure 4-5 Formula to Calculate Prevalence from a 2 × 2 Table.

$$\text{Prevalence} = \frac{A + C}{A + B + C + D}$$

If you administer a screening test with an established sensitivity and specificity in a population with a high prevalence of the disease, your screening will have a heightened positive predictive value. If the population does not have a high prevalence of the disease, PPV is decreased. Even without looking at the 2 × 2 table, this phenomenon makes intuitive sense. If you are looking for a disease that is very rare, a positive test result in that population is more likely to be a false positive than in a population where 90% of the population actually has the disease.

Negative Predictive Value

A related concept is the **negative predictive value (NPV)** of a test: If your subject screens negatively, NPV tells you what the probability is that the patient really does not have the disease. Like PPV, this measure depends on sensitivity, specificity, and the prevalence of the illness in the population where you are administering the test. Using the 2 × 2 table again, you can determine the NPV using the equation in Figure 4-6.

Efficiency

One last concept is particularly useful in a clinical setting. **Efficiency (EFF)** is a measure of the agreement between the screening test and the actual clinical diagnosis. To determine efficiency, add all the true positives and all the true negatives and determining what proportion of your sample that is (this is the group the test correctly identified and therefore, the diagnosis is made correctly. That is always a good thing in nursing!) Efficiency can be calculated by using the formula in Figure 4-7.

Summary

You have completed Chapter 4 and are doing a great job! Let's recap the main ideas.

Validity is the accuracy of your measurement. To assess content validity, determine the relevant variables from a thorough literature search, include them in your measurement instrument, and have your instrument reviewed by experts for feedback. For convergent validity, you compare your results with those of another previously validated survey that measured the same thing. Divergent validity is the opposite: It measures the opposite variable of a previously validated measurement and finds the opposite result.

Reliability tells you whether your measurement tool is consistent or repeatable. Stability is one of the main factors that contributes to

Figure 4-6 Formula to Calculate Negative Predictive Value (NPV) from a 2 × 2 Table.

$$NPV = \frac{\text{True negatives (D)}}{\text{All the subjects who tested negative (C + D)}}$$

Figure 4-7 Formula for Calculating Efficiency (EFF).

$$EFF = \frac{A + D}{A + B + C + D} \times 100$$

reliability and is the consistent or enduring quality of the measure. Another component or type of reliability is homogeneity or the extent to which items on a multi-item instrument are consistent with each other. Also, equivalence reliability tells you if multiple forms or multiple users of an instrument produce the same results.

Nurses like to know the sensitivity and specificity of screening tests. Sensitivity is the probability of getting a true positive, and specificity is the probability of getting a true negative.

Prevalence of the illness in a population affects the positive and negative predictive values of a screening test.

Again, great work for completing this difficult chapter. If you are somewhat confused by these new concepts, continue to practice, practice, practice! Believe it or not, you will look back on these concepts at the end of the semester, and they will make sense. For those of you who feel comfortable with these new concepts, continue to Chapter 5. You're almost half way there!

CHAPTER 4 REVIEW QUESTIONS

1. Your test is very good at correctly identifying when a person actually has a disease. This is a measure of:

   a. sensitivity.

   b. specificity.

   c. collinearity.

   d. effect size.

2. If a person has a disease and tests positive for it, the result is an example of a:

   a. true negative.

   b. false positive.

   c. false negative.

   d. true positive.

Questions 3–4: You are studying a new screening test. Of the 100 people who do not have a disease, 80 test negative for it with your new screen. Of the 100 people who do have the disease, 90 test positive with your screen.

   3. The sensitivity of your screen is _____.

   4. Your new screen's specificity is _____.

5. You have a new tool that examines outcomes in pregnancy. A previously validated tool reports that cesarean section rates in your area are 30%. The correlation between the old tool and your tool is 0.7. This result indicates:

    a. convergent validity.

    b. content validity.

    c. divergent validity.

    d. validity from contrasting groups.

Questions 6–13: You are developing a new screening test and construct the test results shown in Figure 4-8.

Figure 4-8 2 × 2 Table.

	Disease Present	Disease Not Present	Totals
Test positive	44	3	47
Test negative	6	97	103
Totals	50	100	150

6. How many true positives do you have?

7. Explain in English what each box represents.

8. What is the sensitivity of your new test?

9. What is the specificity of your new test?

10. Give an example of a clinical situation in which this might be a good test to use.

11. What is the positive predictive value of your screening test?

(continues)

12. What is the prevalence of the disease you are testing for?

_____

13. If this disease is fatal would you be concerned about this prevalence rate?

_____

Research Application

Questions 14–17: A small study was done to compare the results from three different Chlamydia screening tests. The results obtained are shown in Figure 4-9.

Figure 4-9 2 × 2 Table for Chlamydia Screen.

	Sensitivity	Specificity	PPV	NPV
Screen A	57	96	66	94
Screen B	85	82	37	98
Screen C	57	94	57	94

14. Which screen has the lowest specificity? Why might it still be a good screen to use?

_____

_____

15. Which screen has the highest positive predictive value? If you administered this screen in a population with a high prevalence, what would you expect to happen to the positive predictive value?

_____

_____

16. If you know that early treatment helps prevent infertility and that chlamydia is very contagious, would sensitivity or specificity be more important to you? With that in mind, which of these tests would you prefer to utilize?

_____

_____

17. If all the tests are administered in the same manner and cost the same, which one would you recommend that your clinic use? Justify your answer.

_____

_____

Questions 18–23: You are using a screening test in your clinic to detect abnormal cervical cells related to the presence of human papilloma virus (HPV). Your results are shown in Figure 4-10.

Figure 4-10 Screening Test Results.

	Abnormal Cells Present	Abnormal Cells Not Present	Totals
Test positive	360	20	380
Test negative	40	80	120
Totals	400	100	500

18. What is the prevalence of abnormal cells in your clinic? What does this mean in English?

_____

19. What is the sensitivity of the screen? What does this mean in English?

_____

20. What is the specificity of the screen? What does this mean in English?

_____

21. What is the positive predictive value of the screen (PPV)? What does this mean in English?

_____

22. What is the negative predictive value of the screen (NPV)? What does this mean in English?

_____

23. What is the efficacy of the screen? What does this mean in English?

_____

(continues)

Questions 24–31: A new vaccine is developed that provides immunity to the virus causing abnormal cervical cells, and you reexamine data two years after the vaccine is implemented at your clinic. See the results in Figure 4-11.

Figure 4-11 Screening Test Results After Vaccine Implementation.

	Abnormal Cells Present	Abnormal Cells Not Present	Totals
Test positive	180	60	240
Test negative	20	240	260
Totals	200	300	500

24. What is the prevalence of abnormal cervical cells after the vaccine is utilized? How did the vaccine affect the prevalence?

_____

_____

25. What is the sensitivity of the screen? Does a change in prevalence affect the sensitivity?

_____

_____

26. What is the specificity of the screen? Does a change in prevalence affect the specificity?

_____

_____

27. What is the positive predictive value (PPV) of the screen? Does a change in prevalence affect the PPV? How?

_____

_____

28. What is the negative predictive value (NPV) of the screen? Does a change in prevalence affect the NPV? How?

_____

_____

29. What happens to the number of false positives when the prevalence rates go down?

_____

_____

30. What happens to the efficacy of the screen when prevalence rates go down?

_____

_____

31. Why might you consider lengthening the time between screens or developing a more specific screen with the new prevalence rate?

_____

_____

ANSWERS TO CHAPTER 4 REVIEW QUESTIONS

1. A

3. 90%

5. A

7. 44 = true positives, 3 = false positives, 47 = all positive tests, 6 = false negatives, 97 = true negatives, 103 = all negative tests, 50 = total with disease, 100 = healthy total, 150 = total population

9. 97 ÷ 100 = 97%

11. 44 ÷ 47 = 93.6%

13. Yes! A third of the population has the disease. That is a substantial disease burden.

15. A, high prevalence increases PPV; therefore, the PPV would increase.

17. Answers will vary, but should not include screen C, which has lower specificity and PPV than screen A and the same sensitivity and NPV.

19. 360 ÷ 400 = 90% (If the patient has abnormal cervical cells, there is a 90% probability that the screen will be positive and detect the abnormal cells.)

21. 360 ÷ 380 = 94.7% (Of all the patients who screen positive, 94.7% are patients who really have abnormal cervical cells.)

(continues)

23. $440 \div 500 = 88\%$ (Eighty-eight percent of the time the screen correctly identifies the patient's disease state.)

25. $180 \div 200 = 90\%$ (stays the same)

27. $180 \div 240 = 75\%$ (PPV decreases when prevalence goes down! You are more likely to have false positives in areas with lower prevalence.)

29. False positives increase.

31. Answers will vary but should include: False positives create a financial burden because unnecessary services are provided. Also there may be negative health impacts from the stress, anxiety, loss of work time, and any other unnecessary screens or procedures that result from the false positive screen.

Sampling Methods

Does the sample represent the population?

OBJECTIVES

By the end of this chapter students will be able to:

- Compare and contrast probability and non-probability sampling, and describe at least one example of each.

- Identify similarities and differences among simple random sampling, systematic sampling, stratified sampling, and cluster sampling.

- Identify sampling error, contrast it with sampling bias, and identify the effect of each.

- Explain why the central limit theorem is useful in statistics.

- Identify situations in which nonprobability sampling is utilized and what limits are created by doing so.

- Given a research proposal, compose inclusion and exclusion criteria.

- Evaluate sampling techniques strengths and weakness in a current research article.

KEY TERMS

Cluster sampling
Probability sampling using a group or unit rather than an individual.

Convenience sampling
A form of nonprobability sampling that consists of collecting data from the group that is available.

Exclusion criteria
The list of characteristics that would eliminate a subject from being eligible to participate in your study.

Inclusion criteria
The list of characteristics a subject must have to be eligible to participate in your study.

Nonprobability sampling
Involves methods in which subjects do not have the same chance of being selected for participation.

Probability sampling
Techniques in which the probability of selecting each subject is known.

Quota sampling
A form of nonprobability sampling done when you select the proportions of the sample for different subgroups, much the same as in stratified sampling but without random selection.

Sampling bias
A systematic error made in the sample selection that results in a non-random sample.

Sampling distribution
All the possible values of a statistic from all the possible samples of a given population.

Sampling error
Differences between the sample and the population that occur due to randomization or chance.

Sampling method
The processes employed to select the subjects for a sample from the population being studied.

Simple random sampling
Probability sampling in which every subject in a population has the same chance of being selected.

Stratified sampling
Probability sampling that divides the population into subsamples according to a characteristic of interest and then randomly selects the sample from these subgroups.

Systematic sampling
Probability sampling involving the selection of subjects according to a standardized rule.

Sampling Methods

Let's revisit the original concepts of populations and samples. A population is the whole group that is of interest to the researcher. For example, all men with heart disease are a population. However, although you are amazing as a nurse

researcher, measuring the life spans of all men with heart disease is impossible. Instead, you decide to collect a representative sample of these men. To be representative of the population, the sample must reflect its important characteristics. For example, if 50% of men who have heart disease are over 60 years old, 50% of your sample population should also be men over 60 years old. Your sample, then, is a group of subjects selected from the population for the purpose of conducting your research. Because it is representative, you can then develop inferences about the original population from your sample population.

The **sampling method** you will use consists of the processes of selecting the subjects for your sample from the population under study. Of the many kinds of sampling methods, the one you select depends a great deal on your population of interest and on the options available to you at the time. There are two main kinds of sampling methods: probability sampling and nonprobability sampling.

Probability Sampling

Probability sampling consists of techniques in which the probability of selecting each subject is known. It can be accomplished in a number of ways including: simple random sampling, systematic sampling, stratified sampling, and cluster sampling.

Simple Random Sampling

With **simple random sampling**, every subject in a population has the same chance of being selected. Because this type of sampling requires the researcher to have access to every member of the population, it is frequently not feasible with large populations. However, suppose as the nursing researcher you wish to find out the mean age of the nurses at your hospital. You could use a list of all hospital nurses ($n = 100$) and then randomly select fifty subjects from the list for your sample. As long as selection is from all 100 nurses each time, the probability of selecting each individual is exactly the same (1/100). Although simple random sampling is the ideal, it doesn't work without access to the full population.

Systematic Sampling

A similar approach, **systematic sampling**, involves selecting your subjects according to a standardized rule. One way of doing this is to number the whole population again, pick a random starting point, and then select every *n*th person. For example, you might take the same list of nurses from your hospital and randomly start with the 17th nurse on the list and then select every 9th one. When using this approach, you have to make sure the population list is not developed with any ranking order. For example, if your list is arranged by clinical track levels for each unit, the 9th person may fall into about the same track level consistently, and that may be an achievement related to age. Your sample would then not be representative of the population of nurses working at your hospital.

Stratified Sampling

Stratified sampling divides the population into subsamples according to a characteristic of interest and then randomly selects the sample from these subgroups. The purpose is to ensure representativeness of the characteristic. An example should make that clearer. You are still trying to determine the average age of the nurses in your hospital. You are aware that 20% of the nurses have been practicing for one year or less, and the rest have more than one year of experience. You decide to use stratified random sampling to make sure your sample is representative of the population in terms of working experience. So you decide to select 20% of your sample randomly from the nurses who have one year or less of experience and 80% of your sample from those who have more than one year of experience.

Cluster Sampling

Cluster sampling uses a group or unit rather than an individual. It is used when it is difficult to find a list of the entire population. If, for example, you wanted to know the mean income of adults living in New York State you may choose to survey everyone over age 21 in four randomly selected zip codes and take a weighted average score. Or, if you wanted to know the mean age of nurses employed in hospitals in New York, you may decide to randomly select a sample of hospitals in New York (each hospital is a cluster or group) and then find out the age of all of the nurses at those hospitals.

If that approach is too difficult, you can do two-staged cluster sampling. Rather than taking the age of each nurse at the cluster hospitals, you would randomly sample a group of nurses at each hospital. In effect, you randomly selected your clusters and then randomly selected your final sample from each of these clusters. Although less expensive than other methods, cluster sampling has its drawbacks in terms of statistics as well (greater variance) but is sometimes a necessary approach (Pagano & Gauvreau, 1993).

Sampling Error Versus Sampling Bias

No matter what random sampling technique you choose for your study, there will always be some **sampling error**, that is, some differences between the sample and the population that occur due to chance. Anytime you are examining a random sample and not the whole population, you will encounter some differences that are not under your control and that occur due only to the randomization or chance.

Sampling error, however, is not the same as **sampling bias**, which is a systematic error made in the sample selection that results in a nonrandom sample. In the previous example, you decided to take a systematic sample from a list of nurses at your hospital to determine the mean number of years they worked at your hospital. Unfortunately, you did not realize that the list

was arranged by clinical track levels for each unit. You chose to start at the beginning and sample every 9th person. Unfortunately, the 9th person fell in about the same track level consistently, and track levels are related to the number of years worked at the hospital. Your results would have had a significant amount of sampling bias and would not be representative of the population of interest.

Sampling Distributions

Talking about the benefits of random sampling can get a little statistical, but bear with me. Suppose you collect a *random* sample of nurses from a population of nurses, calculate the mean age, and keep doing this with other random samples of nurses from the same population. Eventually you will develop a distribution of the mean age. This is your **sampling distribution**, which consists of all the possible values of a statistic from all the possible samples of a given population (Corty, 2007). See Figures 5-1 and 5-2.

Figure 5-1 Sampling Distribution for the Mean Age of Nurses.

Sample	Mean Age
One	28
Two	30
Three	30
Four	30
Five	28
Six	26
Seven	32
Eight	32
Nine	34

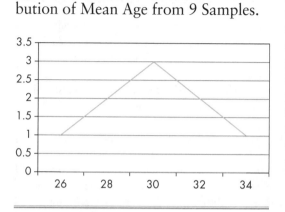

Figure 5-2 Graph of Sample Distribution of Mean Age from 9 Samples.

The really useful thing about sampling distributions is that, if your sample size is large enough (usually at least greater than 30, some say 50), the distribution of the sample means is always normally distributed even if the original population is not (Sullivan, 2007). You can thank the central limit theorem. For the purposes of this introductory class, you don't need to delve too much into the explanation. The takeaway message is that, when a population is not distributed normally, it takes a lot more work to analyze.

FROM THE STATISTICIAN   BRENDAN HEAVEY

The Central Limit Theorem and Standardized Scores

The central limit theorem is your friend. It makes a bunch of analyses a *lot* simpler. It's a little tough to grasp perhaps, but, if you apply yourself just a little bit, you'll be able to pick it up without a problem. Then you can apply it later on anytime you want.

One way to understand the central limit theorem is to see what happens when you roll a bunch of 10-sided dice. You can apply this analogy to *any* random experiment that involves identically likely outcomes.

If we were to roll a 10-sided die 1000 times and plot a histogram of your results, the graph could look something like the one in Figure 5-3. We could get a huge amount of possible bar charts, but they would all look something like the one in the figure. In fact, in the long run this experiment would use what we call the *uniform distribution* because all cases are equally likely. If we were to roll a single die 1000, 2000, or even 10,000 times, all the bars would still look approximately the same.

Now let's think about what would happen if we were to use two 10-sided dice, roll them 1000 times, and calculate the average value shown on the faces. It just so happens I enjoy doing this sort of thing in my spare time; so I went ahead and did so. The result is shown in Figure 5-4. What do you notice? The bars tend to look more bell shaped, don't they? There were a whole lot more results between 4 and 6 than there were 1s and 10s. When you roll two dice, there are a lot more ways to get an average between 4 and 6 than there are to get a 1 or a 10. In fact, the only way to average a 1 is by having both dice come up with 1s!

Now let's look at what happens when we use six 10-sided dice and take the average. The bar graph in Figure 5-5 looks even more bell shaped.

(continues)

FROM THE STATISTICIAN   BRENDAN HEAVEY

This progression demonstrates the central limit theory. In fact, what the underlying distributions look like doesn't matter; you could use a 4-sided die, a 12-sided die, a 6-sided die, or a 20-sided die and plot the outcomes. As you take more and more samples, the resulting distribution of the averages of all the die will tend to look more and more bell shaped!

Remember that we're talking about the mean value of *all* the rolls. You can't just roll a single die a million times and expect it to look more and more bell shaped as you increase the number of rolls. You have to look at the mean value across multiple experiments.

The central limit theorem is one of the most important in all of statistics. It can be proven, but it takes a whole lot of math that I'm sure you don't want to see. We can make some very important and very interesting deductions from this theorem. One is that, when you take a sample in any experiment, the population variables can be distributed in any matter you want, but the mean of the sample measurement will always be distributed as a normal distribution in the long run. This becomes *really* important when we start to look at comparing the means of two samples later on. (Curb your enthusiasm! I know I can't wait!)

Figure 5-3 Central Limit Theorem: One 10-sided Die Rolled 1000 Times.

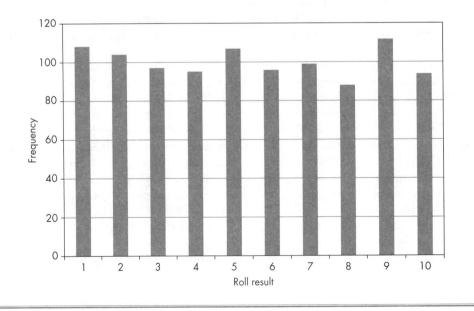

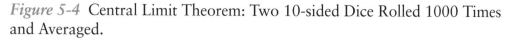

Figure 5-4 Central Limit Theorem: Two 10-sided Dice Rolled 1000 Times and Averaged.

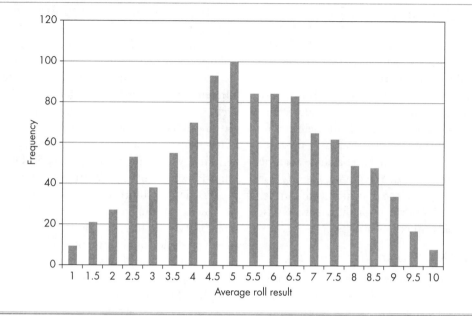

Figure 5-5 Central Limit Theorem: Six 10-sided Dice Rolled and Averaged 1000 Times.

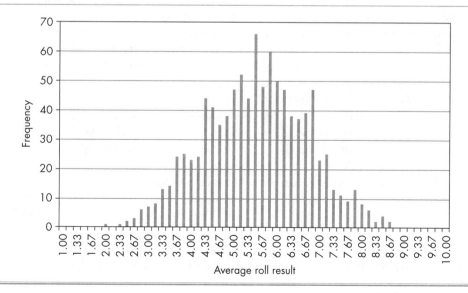

Nonprobability Sampling

The reality of research is that it has budgetary and time limits. In these situations, sometimes nonprobability sampling methods are necessary or simply more practical. **Nonprobability sampling** consists of methods in which subjects do not have the same chance of being selected for participation. It is *not randomized*. When you are reading nursing research, never assume a sample was randomly selected. You need to identify how the sample was selected before you can tell whether the claims the research makes are valid or what their limitations may be.

Types of Nonprobability Sampling

There are many different ways non-probability sampling can be used in both quantitative and qualitative research. Two of the most popular methods for quantitative research are convenience sampling and quota sampling, while qualitative research may employ network sampling or purposive sampling.

CONVENIENCE SAMPLING

The most popular form of nonprobability sampling in healthcare research is **convenience sampling**, which is simply collecting data from the available group. For example, suppose you were trying to determine the mean age of the nurses in your hospital. You go to the oncology unit and ask all the nurses working that shift their age. You would be taking a convenience sample. Convenience samples are usually relatively quick and inexpensive, but they are not representative of the population and therefore limit any inferences you may choose to make about the population.

QUOTA SAMPLING

In **quota sampling**, you select the proportions of the sample for different subgroups, as in strat-ified sampling. For example, if 50% of your population works day shift, 30% works evening shift, and 20% works night shift, your sample will have those same proportions. I bet right now you are thinking, "But this doesn't seem to be different from stratified random sampling." Well, so far—you're right, nothing is different yet. The difference is after this point. If you need a final sample size of 100, with stratified random sampling, you would *randomly* select 50 subjects from day shift workers, 30 from evening shift workers, and 20 subjects from night shift workers. Quota sampling, on the other hand, is nonprobability sampling so it is not randomized. After you decide on the proportions of the sample, you collect subjects continuously until you have 50 day shift subjects, 30 evening shift subjects, and 20 night shift subjects.

Now suppose that you decide to collect this sample at 3:30 in the lobby of your hospital. Everyone who participates gets a free coffee coupon. Fifty day shift nurses participate on their way out, and 30 evening shift nurses participated on their way in. You have enrolled all your day and evening nurses but are still waiting for the night nurses. At 10:45 the night shift nurses start to come through the lobby. As you are surveying the night shift staffers, an evening nurse, ending her shift, comes over and volunteers to participate. You cannot include her because you already have your quota of evening shift nurses and are still collecting only night shift nurses. The evening shift nurse becomes irate because she really wants to be in your study (read "really wants the coffee"), and she calls several of her friends to also come in and volunteer. (Nurses *will* do a lot for free coffee!) They too are upset because they were not working that day and were therefore never given the opportunity to participate. Because they worked the day and evening shifts, they are also not eligible to participate because you have also filled the quotas for these shifts.

You end up sitting in the lobby with several very upset day and evening nurses who don't understand why you can't let them participate, at the same time still asking the night shift nurses to join the study and giving them coffee. "The night shift gets everything!" the other nurses complain. Because you are exceptionally patient and have already had your extra coffee that day, you patiently explain that quota sampling does not give the same opportunity to everyone to participate. You are very sorry. You would love to give everyone free coffee, but you need only night nurses now. This is how quota sampling works. Once you have reached the quota for that particular group no matter how many more subjects from that group arrive you do not enroll them and only collect data from the groups in which you have not met your quota.

Of course, after such a stressful experience you may also decide either to change your sampling method or to go to a different hospital to collect data next time. These nurses are intense!

Nonprobability Sampling in Qualitative Research

Many other nonprobability-based sampling methods are more frequently used with qualitative research. Network sampling, for example, utilizes the social networks of friends and families to gather information. This technique is frequently used when you need information about groups that hesitate to participate in research, such as youth gangs. Another technique, purposive sampling, includes subjects because they have particularly strong bases of information. You may decide to use network sampling to study youth gangs after you are able to gain the trust and support of a gang leader. She then refers other members of her gang to you, and you are able eventually to speak to a group of ten youth gang members. You may then decide to collect a purposive sample (specific individuals are selected to participate because of the information they are able to contribute) and further study three of these young women because they are lifelong gang members and can give you the greatest insight into the characteristics and behaviors you are studying.

Inclusion and Exclusion Criteria

No matter which sampling method you select, as the researcher you need to develop sample inclusion and exclusion criteria.

- **Inclusion criteria** make up the list of characteristics a subject must have to be eligible to participate in your study. These criteria identify the target population and limit the generalizability of your study results to this population. For example, if you are studying the effect of taking a multivitamin on future prostate cancer development, the foremost inclusion criterion is male gender (think about this—only men have prostates so it would be pointless to include women in this study).

- **Exclusion criteria** are the criteria or characteristics that eliminate a subject from being eligible to participate in your study. Exclusion criteria frequently include the current or past presence of the outcome of interest. For example, in your study about the vitamin-mediated prevention of prostate cancer, having prostate cancer would be one of your exclusion criteria. If the subject already has or has had the disease, you can't determine whether the vitamin helps to prevent it.

Summary

That was a lot of information to take in for one chapter. So take a deep breath and allow your brain to slow down! Let's highlight the main ideas.

A sampling method consists of the processes that help you pick the subjects for your sample from the population you are interested in studying. The two main kinds of sampling methods are probability sampling and nonprobability sampling. Probability sampling involves techniques in which the probability of selecting each subject is known. The types of probability sampling include simple random sampling, systematic sampling, stratified sampling, and cluster sampling. Nonprobability sampling involves methods in which subjects do not have the same chance of being selected for participation. In other words, sampling is not randomized. Nonprobability sampling includes convenience sampling, quota sampling, network sampling and purposive sampling.

When you are collecting samples, sampling error can occur; that is, some differences between the sample and the population always occur due to randomization or chance. Sampling bias, however, can also occur, which is the result of a systematic error in the sample selection, rendering it nonrandom.

Finally, all research studies have inclusion and exclusion criteria. Inclusion criteria make up a list of characteristics that a subject must have to participate in your study. Exclusion criteria are the criteria or characteristics that eliminate a subject from being eligible to participate.

You are done with this chapter. Take a break. Drink some tea and unwind a bit! There is more good stuff coming in Chapter 6 when we start to talk about your research ideas!

CHAPTER 5 REVIEW QUESTIONS

1. What is the difference between probability and nonprobability sampling?

_____

_____

2. Identify whether probability or nonprobability sampling was utilized for each entry in the following list:
   a. Convenience sampling
   b. Cluster sampling
   c. Simple random sampling
   d. Quota sampling
   e. Systematic sampling
   f. Stratified sampling

3. What is the difference between sampling error and sampling bias? Which one is very concerning to researchers?

_____

_____

Research Application

Questions 4–5: The study sample was a convenience sample drawn from the clients utilizing two community-based obstetric offices within an area with limited socioeconomic conditions. The sample was drawn largely from the community surrounding the offices and the findings may not be generalizable to this population or other populations which differ significantly from this sample.[*]

4. Why should a reader be careful about developing inferences about the population of interest from the article?

5. How could the researcher have designed this study differently so that it would not be a concern?

6. Hemoglobin levels are usually 12–16 g/100 ml for women and 14–18 g/100 ml for men. If you have a sampling distribution of mean hemoglobin levels (collected from 60 hospitals) with a mean of 16 g/100 ml and a standard deviation of 2 g/100 ml, calculate the range of hemoglobin levels that would include 68% of your sample means.

7. What percentage of sample means would fall between 12 g/100 ml and 20 g/100 ml?

8. If one of the hospitals in your sample was a Veterans Affairs facility with 97% male patients, would you expect the mean the hemoglobin level collected only from the patients at that hospital to be any different from that of other hospitals?

9. If one of the hospitals in your sample was the regional Women's and Children's Hospital, would you expect the mean hemoglobin level collected at that hospital to be different from that of the other hospitals?

*This text is reprinted with the permission of Elsevier and was originally published in Heavey, E., Moysich, K., Hyland, A., Druschel, C., & Sill, M. (2008). Female adolescents' perception of male partners' pregnancy desire. *Journal of Midwifery and Women's Health, 53*(4), 338–344. Copyright Elsevier (2008).

The companion website for this book has a research application article for this material. Check it out!

Answers to Chapter 5 Review Questions

1. With probability sampling, the probability of selecting each subject is known and is the same. With nonprobability sampling, the subjects do not have the same chance of being selected.

3. Sampling error is random error due to chance. Systematic error results in a nonrandom sample and is very concerning to researchers.

5. A randomized sample improves representativeness and expands generalizability.

7. 95% (mean $\pm$ two standard deviations)

9. Yes, hemoglobin levels are lower for women and children.

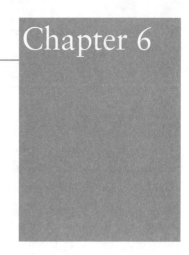

Chapter 6

Generating the Research Idea

What is my research idea?

KEY TERMS

Alpha

The significance level, usually 0.05. The probability of incorrectly rejecting the null hypothesis or making a type one error.

Alternative hypothesis

Usually the relationship or association or difference that the researcher actually believes to be present.

Clinically significant

A result that is statistically significant and clinically useful.

Fail to reject the null hypothesis

When you do not have enough statistical strength to show a difference or association.

Hypothesis

An observation or idea that can be tested.

Hypothesis testing

The application of a statistical test to determine whether an observation or idea is to be refuted or accepted.

Null hypothesis

That there is no difference or association between variables that is any greater or less than would be expected by chance.

Reject the null hypothesis

When you have enough statistical strength to show a difference or association.

Statistical significance

When the difference you observe between two samples is large enough that it is not simply due to chance.

Type one error

Occurs when you incorrectly reject the null hypothesis.

Hypothesis Testing

When you arrive at the clinic at 8 a.m., you are prepared to administer the flu vaccine to patients who show up for one. Already people are waiting, and many are wearing business attire. The turnout is much higher than your clinic expected, processing everyone is taking longer than expected, and you are the only nurse. The patients are brought into a central receiving area, their background information is collected, and then they come to your station for the actual injection. After the first hour you notice that most of your patients are elderly or unemployed. You realize that it is after now after 9 a.m. Very few individuals who report outside employment arrive during the hours of 9 a.m. and 5 p.m. You start to wonder whether employed individuals are less likely to get their flu shots because they are unable to come to the clinic during standard business hours and those who arrived before work may not have been able to stay due to the long delays.

This is a **hypothesis**, an observation or idea that can be tested. You decide to determine whether your observation is actually true. First, you develop your **null hypothesis**, which states that there is no difference or association between variables that is any greater or less than would be expected by chance. (The null hypothesis is represented as H_0.) In this case, the null hypothesis is that there is no relationship between employment status and having a flu shot at your clinic. The **alternative hypothesis** is usually the relationship or association or difference that the researcher actually believes to be present. (The alternative hypothesis is represented as H_1.) In this case, your alternative hypothesis is that those who are employed are less likely to get a flu shot at your clinic: **Hypothesis testing**, a big fancy term for figuring out whether you are right, involves using a statistical test to determine whether your hypothesis is true. In this case, that night when the clinic closes, you decide to collect the information that was gathered on all the patients who arrived at the clinic from 8 a.m. until 9 p.m. that week. This is your sample.

Your statistical analysis of the sample enables you to do one of two things:

- If the trend of having very few employed patients arriving for flu shots at your clinic continued throughout the day, you may find a *statistically significant difference* (we'll tell you how to do this later in the chapter) between the number of employed people who received the flu shot at your clinic that week and those who were not. You are then in a position to **reject the null hypothesis**. You have determined the difference between the two groups is greater than the difference you might expect to result from chance. You have evidence of a statistically significant relationship between employment status and receiving a flu shot at your

clinic, and you have demonstrated support for your alternative hypothesis.
- On the other hand, let's say you collect and analyze the data from the whole week and find that, although there were less employed people receiving flu shots between 9 a.m. and 5 p.m. (your initial impression) between 8 and 9 a.m. and between 5 and 9 p.m., most of the flu shot recipients were employed. In this case, your statistical analysis may not show a significant difference between the number of people who received the flu shot who were employed and those who were not. You would then **fail to reject the null hypothesis**. This is the important point: You can never "accept" or "prove" the null hypothesis, which is the absence of something. You can only "disprove" it (reject it) or fail to "disprove" it (fail to reject it).

Here's an analogy for this slightly confusing concept that obstetrics nurses usually understand fairly quickly so let's use their clinical experience to help you too. When a pregnant patient has an ultrasound, the technician attempts to determine the sex of the infant by detecting the presence of a penis. The null hypothesis is that there is no penis. The alternative hypothesis is that there is one. If a penis is detected, the ultrasound technician can state that there is one and the baby is a boy. If a penis is not detected, the technician *cannot* be sure that there isn't one; it might be present but undetected (Corty, 2007). As a nurse–midwife, I frequently explained to my patients that if the ultrasound technician told them they are carrying a baby boy, they could consider the report fairly reliable (but notice this is still not a probability of 100%). However, I have been in the delivery room when a predicted girl turned out to be a bashful boy. Never overstate what your data allows you to say! You can never say for sure that something does not exist, but the mere presence of what you are looking for can demonstrate that it does. That being said, it is also important to remember that statistics is all about probability and there is always a possibility of an error so you can never "prove" anything with absolute certainty. The technician who thinks she sees a baby boy could still just be wrong!

Statistical Significance

Statistical significance means that the difference you observe between two samples is large enough that it is not simply due to chance. We are going to talk a lot in this book about statistical significance; it is a key concept. There are many different ways to show statistical significance but the basic idea remains the same: If you take two or more representative samples from the same population, you would expect to find approximately the same difference again and again. If you have a statistically significant result, you can reject the null hypothesis.

But how do you know whether your result is statistically significant? At the beginning of the study, the researcher selects the significance level, or **alpha**, which is usually 0.05. This number is simply the probability assigned to incorrectly rejecting the null hypothesis, or to making what is called a **type one error**. For example, you conduct a study examining the association between eating a high-fiber breakfast and 10-a.m. serum glucose levels. The null hypothesis is that a high-fiber breakfast is not associated with the 10-a.m. serum glucose levels. The alternative is that it is. You select an alpha of 0.05. In other words, the alpha of 0.05 means you are accepting that there is a 5% chance that you will reject the null hypothesis incorrectly and report that eating a high-fiber breakfast is associated with a change in blood sugar levels at 10 a.m. when in actuality it is not.

The alpha is therefore the chance of reporting a statistically significant difference that does not exist. An alpha of 0.05 can also be interpreted to mean that you are 95% sure that the significant difference you are reporting is correct.

Corresponding to the alpha (α) is what statisticians call the *p*-value, the probability of observing a value of a test statistic if the null hypothesis (there is no relationship, association or difference between the variables) is true. In other words, a *p*-value tells you the probability of finding your test statistic if there is no relationship between the variables. This is also the probability that an observed relationship, association or difference is just due to chance. For example, if your study examining the consumption of a high fiber breakfast and 10 a.m. glucose levels has a test statistic with a *p*-value of 0.03 then the probability that the observations in your study would occur if there was no relationship between these variables (or by chance) is only 3%. This means you are 97% sure that the variables in your study do have a relationship. If your study has an alpha of 0.05 it means you accept up to a 5% chance of making a type one error and reporting that a relationship exists when it is just by chance. If your test statistic shows you have only a 3% chance of making a type one error then you can confidently reject the null hypothesis and state there is relationship, association or difference between the variables. If the *p*-value is less than the alpha, the researcher should reject the null hypothesis. If it is greater, the chance of making a type one error is too great, and the researcher must fail to reject the null hypothesis. Subtracting the *p*-value from one tells you how sure the statistician is about rejecting the null hypothesis (i.e., A *p*-value of 0.03 means you are 97% sure that the observed relationship is not just due to chance).

FROM THE STATISTICIAN   BRENDAN HEAVEY

Alpha of 0.05: Standard Convention Versus Experiment Specific

Interpreting *p*-values can be a science in and of itself. Let me share with you how I think of *p*-values.

Think about your favorite courtroom drama. Whether you recall OJ Simpson's trial, *A Few Good Men*, *To Kill a Mockingbird*, or *Erin Brockovich*, in all these situations, the defendants are innocent until proven guilty. Therefore, the null hypothesis in these "experiments" is that the defendant is innocent. At all these trials, a defendant is declared not guilty, never innocent. The trial is being conducted—like an experiment—to determine whether to reject the null hypothesis. The null hypothesis cannot be proven; it can only be disproven.

In OJ's case, a lot of people thought there was enough evidence to reject the null hypothesis of innocence and find him guilty. However, as in any criminal case, OJ had to be declared guilty beyond a reasonable doubt. This is a very stringent criterion. Later, in the civil case, the district attorney only had to show a preponderance of evidence to have him declared guilty, which was a much easier task. So OJ was found not guilty in the criminal trial, but guilty in the civil trial. This split decision is the equivalent of different alpha levels determining statistical significance in statistical experiments. The courts reduced the stringency of the test to determine guilt by reducing the burden of proof necessary to convict in a civil trial. Scientists can do the same thing in statistical tests by increasing alpha (which "decreases the burden of proof" in your study). Notice that showing a defendant is guilty in a civil trial (due to a preponderance of evidence) is easier to do than showing he or she is guilty in a criminal trial (beyond a reasonable doubt). Think of a statistical test the same way. If your *p*-value is 0.07 you would reject the null hypothesis if your alpha is 0.10 (less stringent) but not if your alpha is 0.05 (more stringent). It is easier to reject the null hypothesis at the 0.10 level than the 0.05 level.

Note that 0.05 is a very arbitrary alpha cutoff. It has persisted to this day only because R.A. Fisher preferred it, and he's one of the most important statisticians and scientists of all time. He started the practice back in the 1920s, and it has stuck ever since. However, at times scientists use a more stringent cutoff of 0.01 or a less stringent one of 0.1. It's a sliding scale to determine statistical significance, just like the sliding scale of burden of proof in the courtroom!

Statistical Significance Versus Clinical Significance

Statistically significant differences are not the same as clinically significant differences. **Clinically significant differences** are large enough to indicate a preferential course of treatment or a difference in clinical approach to patient care. To be clinically significant, a result must be statistically significant *and* clinically useful. Results that are statistically significant are not necessarily clinically significant, which is a more subjective conclusion.

For example, as a nurse manager, you are approached by the largest chocolate sales team in your region. They say that the newest research shows that patients who receive free chocolate from the hospital are discharged earlier. Well, you might be interested in reading the study. The chocolate team conducted a study with 700,000 participants and found that those who were given free chocolate went home on average 2 minutes earlier than those who didn't.

Although you know chocolate makes people feel better, you do not see these statistically significant results as being clinically significant because a saving of 2 minutes has very little impact on your unit. Besides, what do the follow-up studies say about tooth decay? (We will also talk in the next chapter about how having a very large sample size [700,000 people] in a study might result in statistical significance even though the difference found [the effect size] is actually very small. Stay tuned for that exciting topic!)

FROM THE STATISTICIAN   BRENDAN HEAVEY

Statistical Testing

What if we want to use the information we collect to make informed decisions? What if we want to use the data to decide how to treat patients or how to predict who will most benefit from new treatments? Questions like these make up the core of hypothesis testing. This FTS is a little more difficult, but it is at the very heart of the statistical science presented in this book; so try to hang in there with me.

Most statistical testing procedures can be broken down into the five steps shown in Figure 6-1. A hypothesis test is like a funnel that sorts a whole bunch of information in the form of sample data and decision rules and then spits out a single, easy-to-understand *p*-value. Isn't it great that there is an easy-to-understand answer after all that work?!

The first two steps in a hypothesis test are relatively straightforward, and you already know how to do them. First, you state your null and alternative hypothesis; then you pick the significance level (alpha) that you wish to have in your study. Typically, the alpha is 0.05, which means that, if you find a difference, you are 95% sure it is truly there, not just a chance occurrence).

The *p*-value is related to the alpha. It is just a probability statement about the research. Just as probability ranges between 0 and 1, so do *p*-values. The closer a *p*-value gets to 1, the more likely the related event is (in this case, the conclusion). The closer the *p*-value gets to 0, the less likely it is. Piece of cake, right?

Choosing which statistical test to perform is more difficult, and as you progress in this book you will learn about the many options. Which test you choose depends on a number of things, but usually the most important are how many samples will be compared, how many parts of the population will be estimated, and the format of the variables.

The different forms of statistical tests have a lot in common, though; so we can speak about them in general terms. The tests we discuss in this book all involve computing a so-called "test statistic. One type of test statistic is a *z*-score, which is simply a test statistic that is a standardized measure in a normal distribution. A *z*-score tells you how many standard deviations the observation is from the mean. For example, if $z = 3.4$, the observation is 3.4 standard deviations above the mean score. If $z = -0.2$, then the observation is 0.2 standard deviations below the mean score. A *z*-score, like any other test statistic you compute, has a corresponding *p*-value, which is then used to make the decision to reject or fail to reject the null hypothesis. But where do these *p*-values come from?

Figure 6-2 is a picture of a prototypical hypothesis test using the normal distribution. We can see that the area under the normal curve varies when drawing vertical lines at different *z*-scores. This area is what we need to know in order to report *p*-values. In this case, 2.5% of the probability can be found in each tail of the distribution. The area underneath the normal curve, above the horizontal axis, and to the

FROM THE STATISTICIAN

BRENDAN HEAVEY

outside of our vertical lines totals 0.05 (0.025 in each tail). These vertical lines represent the z-value that corresponds with these probability levels. In this case, the z-value of 2 or -2 is greater than 1.96 (the cut-off for statistical significance on the horizontal axis); so our statistical test falls in the upper tail of the null distribution. Whenever that happens, we say that the observed data is significantly different from what we would expect under the null distribution. Therefore, we conclude this observed difference is not just due to sampling error or chance, and we reject the null hypothesis.

So you should be able to figure out the big question: How much area is under the whole curve in the normal distribution? The answer is 1 or 100% of the probability. As your observation gets farther and farther away from the mean, two things happen:

- The z-score gets pushed farther and farther into the tails of the statistical distribution.
- The p-value associated with that z-score gets smaller and smaller.

And, as you already know, the smaller the p-value is, the less likely it is that this observation is just due to chance and the more sure you are that the difference you found is actually there! You should now be able to understand the link between z-scores and p-values This concept directly transfers from z-scores to t-scores, f-scores, and chi-squared scores which we will discuss in upcoming chapters of this book. Those tests differ in the types of data involved as well as in the quantities being estimated, but they work on this same principle. If the p-value associated with the computed test statistic is less than the alpha value chosen in the decision rule, we should reject the null hypothesis.

Figure 6-1 Hypothesis Testing Steps.

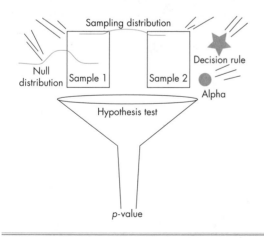

Hypothesis Testing Steps

1. State the null and alternative hypotheses.
2. **Significance level**—Determine what alpha to use to determine statistical significance.
3. **Statistical test**—Determine what statistical test to use.
4. Compare the distribution of the statistic computed in step 3 to the distribution under the null hypothesis and report a p-value.
5. **Decision rule**—Decide whether to reject the null hypothesis or not (Is the sample distribution different enough from the null distribution to say it is more than a chance occurrence?).

Figure 6-2 The Normal Curve.

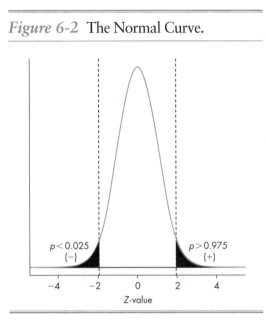

is no relationship, association or difference. The alternative hypothesis is the opposite of the null: There is a relationship, association or difference (what you actually think is true). Hypothesis testing involves using a sample to determine whether your hypothesis is true.

When you reject the null hypothesis, you have found statistical support for your alternative hypothesis. When you fail to reject the null hypothesis, you do not have enough statistical strength to say there is a relationship or association. There may not really be a relationship, or you may not have a sample that is large enough (we will talk about this more in the next chapter). You can never accept the null hypothesis. If you reject the null hypothesis incorrectly, it is a type one error.

Statistical significance means that the difference you observed between two samples is large enough that it is not simply due to chance. To determine statistical significance, you need to identify a significance level, called the alpha, which is usually 0.05. If your p-value is less than alpha, you have statistical significance. For something to be clinically significant, a result must be statistically significant and clinically useful.

This chapter presented a lot of information, but if you are able to grasp these concepts, you are doing well! Don't worry. We will continue to work with these ideas and reinforce them as you build your knowledge!

Summary

You have just completed Chapter 6! The concepts are getting more technical, but keep reviewing and practicing to maintain and enhance your knowledge. Now we can review some of the important concepts in this chapter.

A hypothesis is an observation or idea that can be tested. The null hypothesis states that there

CHAPTER 6 REVIEW QUESTIONS

1. You are conducting a study to determine whether there is an association between years worked in nursing and salary earned. Write the null and alternative hypotheses.

_____

_____

2. If you find a p-value of 0.09, what would you conclude?

_____

3. If you find a p-value of 0.03, what would you conclude?

_____

4. If you reject the null hypothesis, what type of error is it if you are wrong?

_____

5. If your p-value is 0.03, is the conclusion clinically significant?

_____

6. You are conducting a study to determine whether there is an association between a positive toxicology screen for Rohypnol (flunitrazepam) and signs of sexual assault in a sample collected from three large emergency rooms throughout your state. Write the null and alternative hypotheses.

_____

_____

7. As the primary investigator in this study, you realize your results may be utilized in a courtroom setting, and you do not want to make a type I error. Would you prefer an alpha of 0.05, 0.10, or 0.01?

_____

8. Your study includes all individuals who arrive in the three emergency rooms with a diagnosis of sexual assault over a 1-month period. This is what type of sample?

_____

9. You conduct the study with an alpha of 0.05, and your test statistic has a p-value of 0.02. What do you conclude?

_____

(continues)

10. You get the consent of the study participants and conduct a follow-up study in which you interview the family members of the individuals included in your study. This is an example of what type of sampling?

_____

11. You ask the family members to describe the appearance and the manner of the individuals who were assaulted when they were taken to the emergency room. Is this a qualitative or quantitative measurement?

_____

12. You also collect a measure of the patient's sedation provided by the sexual assault nurse examiner. It is on a 5-point scale: 0 for no sedation, 1 for mild sedation, 2 for moderate sedation, 3 for heavy sedation, and 5 for unable to arouse. What level of measurement is this?

_____

_____

13. In your sample of 45 patients, 10 showed no signs of sedation, 12 were mildly sedated, 3 were moderately sedated, 13 were heavily sedated, and 7 were not arousable. What percentage were mild or moderately sedated?

_____

14. What is the median level of sedation?

_____

15. You are putting together a grouped frequencies table and want to categorize these responses as patients showing signs of sedation and those not showing signs of sedation. How many patients showed signs of sedation? What percentage of your sample is this?

_____

_____

The companion website for this book
has a research application article
for this material. Check it out!

ANSWERS TO CHAPTER 6 REVIEW QUESTIONS

1. H_0: There is no relationship between years worked and salary earned.

   H_1: There is a relationship between years worked and salary earned. *Or*: More years worked is related to a higher earned salary.

3. Reject the null. The *p*-value is significant; therefore you conclude that there is a relationship between years worked and salary earned.

5. You do not know. It depends on the clinical judgment of the experts in clinical care. You may be one of them!

7. Alpha of 0.01

9. Reject the null. There is an association between a positive toxicology screen for rohypnol and signs of sexual assault.

11. Qualitative

13. $15 \div 45 = 33.3\%$

15. $35 \div 45 = 77.7$

Chapter 7

Sample Size, Effect Size, and Power

So how many subjects do I need?

OBJECTIVES

By the end of the chapter students will be able to:

- Describe the components of sample size calculation and relate them to each other.

- Interpret the power in a current research study and how it would affect the necessary sample size if it were increased or decreased.

- Recognize a type two error and contrast it with a type one error.

- Estimate the chance of a type two or type one error in a current research article.

- Calculate the anticipated effect size in a study.

KEY TERMS

Alpha
The chance of making a type one error.

Beta (β)
The chance of making a type two error.

Effect size
The extent to which a difference/relationship exists between variables in a population (the size of the difference you are attempting to find).

Power analysis
How sample sizes are calculated.

Power
The ability to find a difference or association when one actually exists.

Type one error
The error made when you incorrectly reject the null hypothesis, when you conclude there is a significant relationship but there really is not.

Type two error
The error made when you accept the null incorrectly, missing an association that is really there (sometimes called a power error because you may not have enough power to find an association that really exists).

Effect Size

You've gotten pretty far in your research. You've noticed clinical associations, examined descriptive data, evaluated the measurement tools, generated a hypothesis, and decided on your sampling method. Now you need to determine how many subjects you will actually need to sample. This decision is largely dependent on the **effect size**, or the size of the difference between group means that exists within the population.

Effect size and sample size are inversely proportional: As one increases, the other decreases. This fact surprises a lot of people, but it's not too difficult to grasp if you think about it. If you are anticipating a large difference (i.e., a strong effect), you may need only a small sample. If you are anticipating a small difference (i.e., weak effect size), you may need to collect a very large sample. The closer the two groups means are to each other in the population, the more information you need to demonstrate they are different.

One way to determine effect size mathematically is to divide the difference between the mean in the experimental group and the mean in the control group by the standard deviation of the control group. Some statisticians prefer to delineate small, medium and large effect sizes based on the statistical procedure being conducted while others use general guidelines such as those that follow (Cohen, 1992). Let's look at an example.

Grove (2007) prefers to use the following values:

- A weak effect size is < 0.3 (or −0.3).
- A moderate effect size is 0.3–0.5 (or −0.3 to −0.5).
- A strong effect size is > 0.5 (or −0.5).

If you want to know how much of an actual difference in means this is, you can multiply the effect size by the standard deviation in the control group. For example, in a study on the effect of an intervention with premature infants, the control group had a standard deviation of 10 days.

- An intervention with a weak effect size would be associated with a decrease of less than 3 days of prematurity (0.3 × 10).
- A moderate effect size would be associated with a decrease of 3–5 days in prematurity (0.3 to −0.5 × 10).

- A decrease in more than 5 days of prematurity would be a large effect size (0.5 × 10).

The size of the sample directly relates to the **power** of the study, or the ability to find a difference when one actually exists. The two concepts are directly proportional, that is, as one increases the other must as well. Power is defined as the likelihood of rejecting the null hypothesis correctly; that is, you say there is a relationship and difference, and you are correct. It is usually considered adequate to have a power of 0.80 or 80% (Munro, 2005).

FROM THE STATISTICIAN   BRENDAN HEAVEY

The Four Pillars of Study Planning

Whenever I plan a study, particularly in deciding on sample size, I like to think of myself as juggling four mysterious balls, which represent:

1. Alpha level
2. Effect size
3. Power
4. Sample size

None of these balls is labeled, but knowing any three enables me to know the fourth without seeing any labels.

We've already defined the **alpha** level: the probability of rejecting H_0 (the null hypothesis) given that it is true. For our present purposes, setting alpha to 0.05 every time is acceptable.

Think of *effect size* as the amount of difference between what was hypothesized in H_0 and what we find in our study. When planning a study, we try to ensure that true differences result in statistical significance, but false differences do not. So the smaller the difference is that we want to detect, the larger the number of cases we need to look at. (Effect size is inversely proportional to sample size.)

How does the researcher decide on the size of the difference to look at? This is not a statistical question; it has to be determined by previous studies or by some other scientific means. This determination can be tricky. Statisticians rely heavily on investigators to provide them with a difference that's clinically important. Determining the degree of difference can be a major undertaking and requires much background research. Sometimes figuring this out takes longer than completing the whole study!

(continues)

FROM THE STATISTICIAN   BRENDAN HEAVEY

The third concept, *power*, is probably the most difficult concept to grasp in any introductory statistics class. Many beginning students have trouble understanding it. You can think of power as the probability of rejecting the null hypothesis when the alternative hypothesis is true. Power depends on the truth of the hypothesis under study and totally ignores what happens when the null hypothesis is true. Other analysis methods (specifically, setting an alpha threshold) take into account when the null hypothesis is true. Power takes the analysis a step further.

Most studies typically consider 80% power as adequate; that is, if the alternative hypothesis is true you have a probability of at least 80% that you will reject the null hypothesis. This standard percentage is based on convention, just like having an alpha of 0.05. To increase power (the probability of rejecting the null when the alternative is true) and maintain the same alpha level (the probability of incorrectly rejecting the null), you need to increase the sample size. In simpler terms, increasing power requires increasing sample size in order to maintain the same alpha level. Power is *directly* proportional to sample size: When sample size increases, power increases. If you want to increase power, increase your sample size.

Sample size (represented as *n*) is the fourth ball juggled in study planning. Statisticians always, always, always want to increase sample size. Increasing sample size is rarely a bad thing. The problem is that increasing sample size usually means increasing the cost of a study; so statisticians use other approaches to decide on an acceptable sample size.

There are two usual ways of planning a study. The first involves defining the desired effect size and then figuring out the sample size needed to achieve the related power. Statisticians usually choose 80% power and then decide whether the study is possible given the required sample size. In other words, the juggler in me:

- Selects alpha (juggled object 1) as 0.05.
- Defines the effect size of interest (juggled object 2).
- Sets power to 80% (juggled object 3).
- This leaves me with one last juggling object, the sample size, which is completely determined by the other three. The equations you will use to make these determinations are determined by the statistical technique you will employ in your study.

I then do a cost/benefit analysis on my final sample size to determine whether the study should be done. For example, if the cost of acquiring the necessary data for an adequately sized sample is $100,000, the researcher has to determine if the benefit associated with the anticipated results will have a value greater than this investment.

Another approach to study planning is to determine what sample size is available and then what effect size is needed to achieve the appropriate power level (again, usually 80%). In this case, alpha is again set to 0.05, sample size is set to our determined limit, and power is set to 80%. That leaves the juggled object of effect size to be figured out, and it can now be determined based on the other three. Finally, the researcher must determine whether the effect size is interesting enough to warrant performing the study (this usually involves a cost/benefit analysis).

For instance, oversupplementation of vitamin A has been shown to cause liver damage. We design a study to determine whether the damage is caused by reduced blood flow to the liver. We have been given a National Institutes of Health award for outstanding merit in clinical research based on our previous work with EpiPens. The award is for $500,000 and must be put toward further research. With this amount, we can enroll 25 subjects in our study ($n = 25$), who will be asked to come to the hospital for four hours, fill out a survey, have bloods drawn, and undergo a PET scan. We set the alpha level at 0.05 and power at 0.8, which we figure will be sufficient to predict an increase of 0.8 ml/min/g of blood flow or higher. Unfortunately, with this size sample, we can detect only a very large difference (i.e., effect size) in blood flow to the liver. By the time patients have that much difference in blood flow to the liver, they will have already exhibited other detectable signs and symptoms of liver disease; so the effect size we could find with this sample size is too large to be clinically useful. We need to be able to find a smaller difference for the results to be clinically useful; specifically, the study would be useful only if we can predict a difference of 0.08 ml/min/g or lower. Detecting this small an effect size requires us to enroll more subjects than we can afford with this grant money. Can you figure out what other factors we might adjust to make this study feasible?

That's the juggling act. These four concepts are all interrelated. Changing one can affect all three of the others. Note that alpha is rarely changed to accommodate lack of funding. Instead, we first reduce power because in the scientific community it is generally worse to give up on answers that might be right than it is to waste time on answers that are probably wrong. We'll look at this reasoning more in depth in the next FTS.

Type Two Error

Any time you make a decision, there is a chance that you will make a mistake (like ordering garlic sushi on a blind date—big mistake!). When your decision involves failing to reject the null hypothesis, you must consider the possibility of a **type two error**, that is, the error made when you fail to reject the null *incorrectly*, missing an association that is really there. These errors usually occur because the sample wasn't large enough and the study therefore didn't have enough power to find a difference that really existed. Hence type two errors are also frequently called power errors.

Any hypothesis test has the risk of committing a type two error. This risk is represented by **beta (β)**. You can calculate your chance of a type two error fairly simply. Given that there really is a relationship or difference between the variables you are examining, you will either correctly identify it (i.e., reject H_0 correctly = power) or you will incorrectly miss it (type two error). Since there is a 100% chance that you will be *either* correct *or* incorrect (pretty much true for all life decisions), you know that:

Power (correctly rejecting H_0) + Beta (chance of making a type two error) = 100%

Therefore, if there is an 80% chance that you are correct and find the relationship (power), the chance of a type two error is 20%.

On a practical basis, the convention is to set beta at 20%. So you can quickly calculate beta by subtracting the power of the study (usually 80%, or 0.80) from one: $1 - 0.80 = 0.20$.

A Quick Review of Type One and Type Two Errors

Type one and type two errors seem relatively straightforward until you start trying to think about the both of them together. Sort them out like this. The life decisions rule is that, no matter what you are deciding, there are usually two outcomes: You are (1) correct or (2) incorrect. (All of the philosopher-students are horrified that I see things this way, but bear with me.) The question that all research studies ask is whether the null hypothesis is true: The two variables have no relationship, difference, or association between them. In actuality it may be true or it may not be true and you can reject or fail to reject the null hypothesis in either of this situations.

If the null hypothesis *really is true* and there is no relationship or difference between the variables, you can conclude one of two things:

- You can fail to reject it. You are *correct* in this situation and the probability of reaching this conclusion is 1 − alpha (usually 0.05) or 95%.

- Or you can reject it. Then you are *incorrect* and are making a type one error. The probability of reaching this conclusion is equal to alpha, usually 5%.

If the null hypothesis *is really not true* and there is a relationship between the variables, you can conclude one of two things:

- You can fail to reject it. In this case, you are *incorrect* and are making a type two error. The probability of doing so is equal to β (usually 0.20 or 20%).
- Or you can reject it *correctly*. The probability of reaching this conclusion is 1 − β (usually 80%), which is also the power of your study.

Getting the two types of errors confused is easy; so thinking of them in terms of the null hypothesis is helpful. If you reject the null *and are incorrect* you are making a type one error. If you fail to reject the null *and are incorrect* you are making a type two error. Of course, if you are already a statistician, you may not need this tip—but the rest of us do get confused sometimes!

FROM THE STATISTICIAN   BRENDAN HEAVEY

Which Error Is Worse? The Lesser of Two Evils

How do we decide how many subjects to enroll for a study? This is a bread-and-butter question for statisticians, and their answer involves a concept that many people don't understand. Often statisticians have to decide whether it's worse to commit a type one error or a type two error. Statisticians can debate the question for hours, but in this country's legal system—as well as in most of the world's scientific community and real-life situations—committing a type one error is definitely worse.

Let me explain that point. In any court case, four different scenarios are possible, just as in the hypothesis test explanation. See Figure 7-1. The U.S. legal system is based on the principal that people are innocent until proven guilty (H_0: The defendant is not guilty). Inherent in that principal is a subprincipal that sending an innocent person to jail is much worse than letting a guilty person walk. This is the reason for such an enormous appeals process and why you cannot be tried twice for the same offense.

FROM THE STATISTICIAN BRENDAN HEAVEY

In statistics we have a similar philosophy:

- We put a hard cap on alpha (the probability of a false positive) of about 0.05.
- We shoot for a power of about 80%.
- So beta, the probability of a false negative, is set around 0.20 (a much more likely outcome than the accepted probability for a false positive).

We do the same thing in statistics that the U.S. court system does; we just charge less per hour than the average lawyer!

Medical researchers play by much the same rules. Often, researchers find sets of genes that they think may be involved in causing cancer or some other debilitating disease. Once they have found a set of interest, the next step is to test all of them simultaneously in groups of control versus cancerous subjects. This research process can involve upward of 50,000 genes in thousands of subjects at once. What would go through your head if you had to decide how to run this large and complex analysis? You would have to sort each gene into one of the four categories from the 2 × 2 table. Most of the genes would have the same expression in both cancerous and control tissue, and you could eliminate them from contention. Beyond that set, you'd have to decide which is worse: rejecting the one lone gene that may be the cause of cancer *or* wasting time sifting through too many genes that don't have anything to do with your analysis question. Obviously, rejecting the right answer is the worse of the two evils. Unfortunately this means that scientists' time gets wasted all too often!

Figure 7-1 Criminal Status and Trial Results.

		Truth	
		Defendant is innocent.	**Defendant is guilty.**
Result of the Trial	Defendant is convicted.	Major problem TYPE ONE ERROR	No problem $1 - \beta$ = power
	Defendant is acquitted.	No problem 1-alpha	Minor problem TYPE TWO ERROR

Sample Size

All these ideas are related in that you need to understand them to determine your sample size. Before you even begin a study, you need to decide how many subjects to sample. That decision depends on the size of the difference you are looking to detect. In other words, the sample size you need should give you adequate power to correctly reject the null hypothesis. **Power analysis** is how sample sizes are calculated. The many different equations for calculating sample sizes depend on the statistical techniques the study utilizes. Luckily for you, these calculations are beyond the scope of this book. (So you have something to look forward to in your next stats class!) However, power analysis involves some central concepts no matter what calculation you are using. The sample size you need in your study depends on the:

- Effect size—the anticipated difference you expect to see.
- How much type one error you can tolerate—alpha, or chances of incorrectly saying there is a difference.

- Power—the ability to detect a difference that really exists.

Even after calculating the necessary sample size, you may need to increase it if you anticipate a large number of dropouts or a high nonresponse rate. For example, many nurses who are asked about their sexual orientation may choose not to respond to that question, leaving you with too small of a sample size to draw any conclusions. Likewise, if you are conducting a study over a long period of time, a number of participants will be lost to follow-up or will be unable to participate for various reasons, such death, illness, relocation, and the like. These factors all need to be considered when calculating the number of subjects to include in a sample.

When a sample size is too small, you have a greater chance of a type two error. If you don't have enough subjects, you may not find a statistical difference even though one exists. However, when the sample is too large, you not only waste time and money, but also you have a greater chance of a type one error. You might find a statistical difference that really isn't there and promote a treatment or course of action that may not be the best option for patients.

FROM THE STATISTICIAN   Brendan Heavey

Methods: Calculating Effect Size by Hand

The most important thing to remember about calculating effect size is to divide by the standard deviation. The difficult part is figuring out which standard deviation to use. If we compare two groups, we can turn to more than three possible standard deviation estimates: one from the first group, one from the second group, or any number of pooled and weighted estimates. Which should you use?

Jacob Cohen (1988) first defined effect size as:

$$\frac{\bar{X}_1 - \bar{X}_2}{\sigma}$$

where
X_1 = mean of sample one
X_2 = mean of sample two
σ = standard deviation

FROM THE STATISTICIAN

However, Cohen didn't define which standard deviation to use. For simplicity's sake, many researchers simply divide by the standard deviation in the control or reference group (Grove, 2007). For those of you who are mathematically inclined, we are going to show you a more representative method. We recommend the following formula for calculating the standard deviation (σ) in an effect size calculation (Cohen, 1988):

$$\sigma = \sqrt{\frac{(n_1 - 1)s_1^2 + (n_2 - 1)s_2^2}{n_1 + n_2 - 2}}$$

where

n_1 = observed values from group one
s_1 = standard deviation in the first group
n_2 = observed values from group two
s_2 = standard deviation in the second group

For example, consider two comparisons.

Here's the first comparison. Ten samples of prostate-specific antigen levels were taken in two groups of men: one set of controls and one set who have colorectal cancer. Here's the data:

PSA Results in Colorectal Cancer Study

Control (ng/mil)	Cancer (ng/mil)
1.4	6.2
3.2	7.5
3.5	7.5
2.1	6.7
3.2	9.2
3.3	8.8
2.1	5.7
4.2	8.5
2.2	4.6
3.7	7.9

Here are the effect size calculations in this group work. Referring to Cohen's formula, calculate the mean of sample one (X_1):

$$\bar{X}_1 = \frac{1.4 + 3.2 + 3.5 + 2.1 + 3.2 + 3.3 + 2.1 + 4.2 + 2.2 + 3.7}{10} = \frac{28.9}{10} = 2.89$$

$$SD_1 = \sqrt{\frac{\sum_{i=0}^{n}(X_i - \bar{X})^2}{n-1}}$$

$$= \sqrt{\frac{(1.4 - 2.89)^2 + (3.2 - 2.89)^2 + (3.5 - 2.89)^2 + (2.1 - 2.89)^2 + (3.2 - 2.89)^2 + (3.3 - 2.89)^2 + (2.1 - 2.89)^2 + (4.2 - 2.89)^2 + (2.2 - 2.89)^2 + (3.7 - 2.89)^2}{10 - 1}}$$

$$= 0.89$$

(continues)

Now calculate the mean of sample two (X_2):

$$\bar{X}_2 = \frac{6.2 + 7.5 + 7.5 + 6.7 + 9.2 + 8.8 + 5.7 + 8.5 + 4.6 + 7.9}{10} = \frac{72.6}{10} = 7.26$$

$$SD_2 = \sqrt{\frac{\sum_{i=0}^{n}(X_i - \bar{X})^2}{n-1}}$$

$$= \sqrt{\frac{(6.2-7.26)^2 + (7.5-7.26)^2 + (7.5-7.26)^2 + (6.7-7.26)^2 + (9.2-7.26)^2 + (8.8-7.26)^2 + (5.7-7.26)^2 + (8.5-7.26)^2 + (4.6-7.26)^2 + (7.9-7.26)^2}{10-1}}$$

$$= 1.46$$

Finally, what is the standard deviation?

$$\sigma = \sqrt{\frac{(10-1)(0.89)^2 + (10-1)(1.46)^2}{10+10-2}} = \sqrt{\frac{7.13 + 19.18}{18}} = 1.21$$

Now we can plug the values into the Cohen formula:

$$\text{Effect size} = \frac{\bar{X}_1 - \bar{X}_2}{\sigma} = \frac{2.89 - 7.26}{1.21} = -3.61$$

Now that's a whole lot of calculations to do by hand, and that is why all statistical programming packages will do the work for you.

Here's the second comparison. Make sure to understand what happens when σ (the overall standard deviation measure) increases or decreases. For instance, consider the PSA scores from a follow-up trial to the previous study:

Follow-Up PSA Levels

Control (ng/mil)	Cancer (ng/mil)
3.0	7.0
2.9	7.1
2.8	7.1
3.2	6.9
3.1	6.8
3.0	7.2
3.2	7.1
3.1	6.9
2.9	7.0
2.9	6.9

FROM THE STATISTICIAN BRENDAN HEAVEY

In this trial, we have the following results:

$$\bar{X}_1 = 3.01 \qquad S_1 = 0.137$$

$$\bar{X}_2 = 7.00 \qquad S_2 = 0.125$$

$$\sigma = 0.13$$

$$\text{Effect size} = -30.69$$

So you can see that in the second trial the overall standard deviation was drastically reduced. Despite a relatively small change in the difference between means, we get a drastically changed effect size. In fact, sometimes the difference between means may be smaller in an experiment with a larger overall effect size just because of a smaller standard deviation. This tells us that overall effect and standard deviation are inversely proportional. Can you determine whether the size of the difference between means is directly or indirectly proportional to overall effect size? We will revisit this question in the review exercises at the end of the chapter.

You can also see that sometimes an effect size is negative. What does a negative effect size mean? It tells you the direction of the change. If the effect size is negative, the second group has a larger mean than the first—that's all. Concentrate on the overall magnitude of the change because that is the most important part.

Summary

Way to go! You have completed Chapter 7. Now a quick review.

- The effect size is the extent to which a difference/relationship exists between the variables under study in the population. It is also the size or difference you are attempting to find in your study.
- The power of the study is the ability to find a difference when one actually does exist.
- A power analysis is how sample sizes are actually calculated.

- A type one error is when you reject the null hypothesis and are incorrect. In other words, you stated that there was a difference in the variable when there really was not.
- A type two error is when fail to reject the null incorrectly meaning you miss a relationship that does exist.
- Beta is another name for the chance of committing a type two error.
- The sample size you need in your study depends on the effect size or the anticipated difference you expect to see.

Another job well done! Move on to Chapter 8.

CHAPTER 7 REVIEW QUESTIONS

You are asked to develop a study for a pharmaceutical company to determine whether taking one tablet of drug A is related to lower total cholesterol levels.

1. What is your independent variable?

_____

2. What is your dependent variable?

_____

3. How could you measure your dependent variable quantitatively?

_____

   a. Would this be a continuous or categorical variable?

_____

   b. What level of measurement would this variable be?

_____

4. How could you measure your dependent variable qualitatively?

_____

   a. Would this be a continuous or categorical variable?

_____

   b. What level of measurement would this variable be?

_____

5. You chose to measure taking one tablet of drug A as a yes/no question.
   a. What level of measurement is this variable?

_____

   b. What would be the best measure of central tendency?

_____

6. Write a null hypothesis for your study:

_____

_____

_____

7. Write an alternative hypothesis for your study:

   _____

   _____

   _____

8. If you select an alpha of 0.05 and a power of 80%, what does your decision mean?

   _____

   _____

   _____

9. Your study has an alpha of 0.05, your statistical test determines that the p-value for the relationship between taking one tablet of drug A daily and lowering cholesterol is 0.02. What do you conclude?

   _____

   _____

   _____

10. If your conclusion was actually a type one error, what do you know about taking drug A and cholesterol levels?

   _____

   _____

   _____

11. Based on the preliminary pilot study you conducted, the drug company decides to fund a large-scale clinical trial. This trial results in a p-value of 0.07. What is your conclusion?

   _____

   _____

   _____

12. You determine after the trial that the actual effect size from the medication was smaller than you initially thought. Knowing this, you conclude you may have made what type of error in your conclusion?

   _____

(continues)

13. What was the most likely cause of this error?

_____

_____

14. If your study had an alpha of 0.05 and a power of 80%, calculate the chance that you made a type II error.

_____

_____

15. In each of the following instances, identify which type of error is potentially being made: type one or type two.

a. Your study concludes that ambulation post-op day one from hip replacement surgery is associated with shorter hospital stays.

b. Your study examining the relationship between head trauma and grand mal seizures has an alpha of 0.10 and a beta of 0.80. Your statistical analysis reports a *p*-value of 0.06.

c. Your study finds no relationship between vitamin E consumption and skin cancer.

d. Your original intention was to enroll 500 subjects in your study but only 256 completed both a pre- and post-test. You are concerned about what type of error?

e. Your study has an alpha of 0.05 and a beta of 0.90. You examine a sample of circus workers to determine whether they have higher levels of lung cancer. Your statistical analysis finds a *p*-value of 0.04.

f. The poorly designed pilot studies examining the relationship between mold exposure and asthma and reports a small effect size. You recruit a large sample to attempt to enable your research team to successfully detect this effect size. Having a larger sample size increases the risk of making what type of error?

16. You have two samples of adults preparing for barium enema tests the next day. The control group consumes 2 oz of milk of magnesia with a mean average of 120 ml and a standard deviation of 10 ml of water. The second group is advised to consume more water with their milk of magnesia, and they average 124 ml with a standard deviation 12 ml of water. Calculate the effect size in this experiment. Is it small, moderate, or large by Grove's standards?

CHAPTER 7 FTS REVIEW QUESTIONS

1. Fill in the three empty cells of the following table with A or B:

   A = *X* is directly proportional to *Y* [when *X* goes up, so does *Y*].

   B = *X* is inversely proportional to *Y* [when *X* goes up, *Y* goes down].

X	Y Effect Size	Power
Power	_____	
Sample Size	_____	_____

2. Fill in the the cells of the following table with A or B:

   A = *X* is directly proportional to *Y* [when *X* goes up, so does *Y*]

   B = *X* is inversely proportional to *Y* [when *X* goes up, *Y* goes down]

X	Y Effect Size
Size of difference between means	_____
Overall standard deviation	_____

ANSWERS TO CHAPTER 7 REVIEW QUESTIONS

1. Drug A

3. Serum cholesterol, (a) continuous, (b) interval/ratio

5. (a) nominal, (b) mode

7. Answers may vary: Example: Taking Drug A is associated with a change in cholesterol level. Or: Drug A lowers cholesterol level.

9. Reject the null hypothesis. There is a relationship between taking drug A and cholesterol levels.

11. Fail to reject the null; there is not enough evidence to show a relationship between drug A and cholesterol levels.

13. Inadequate power due to two small of a sample to detect this effect size

15. a. Reject the null, may be a type one error.
    b. Reject the null, may be a type one error.
    c. Fail to reject the null, may be a type two error.
    d. Fail to reject the null, may be a type two error due to inadequate sample.
    e. Reject the null, may be a type one error.
    f. Reject the null, may be a type one error.

ANSWER TO CHAPTER 7 FTS REVIEW QUESTION

1.

	Y	
X	**Effect Size**	**Power**
Power	B inversely proportional	XXXXXXX
Sample Size	B inversely proportional	A directly proportional

Chi-Square

Is there a difference?

OBJECTIVES

By the end of the chapter students will be able to:

- Identify conditions under which the chi-square test is appropriate.

- Identify the question the chi-square test is designed to answer.

- Formulate a null and an alternative hypothesis.

- Formulate a 2 × 2 table from an existing data set.

- Interpret an SPSS printout of a chi-square test and determine what action to take with regard to the null hypothesis. Justify this decision in statistically correct terminology.

- Identify a current research article that uses a chi-square test, and determine the level of measurement of the variables used, if the results are statistically significant, and utilize this information to draw a statistical conclusion.

- Debate whether clinical recommendations should be made from a research article's conclusion. Prepare a public health report using this information.

KEY TERMS

Chi-square (X^2)
A test used with independent samples of nominal- or ordinal-level data.

Degrees of freedom (df)
The number values which are "free to be unknown."

Null hypothesis
Means that there is no relationship/association, or difference.

Chi-Square (X^2) Test

You've covered much ground and prepared well to get to this point, and now you can begin an analysis. Recall that, in most experiments, the **null hypothesis** is that there is no relationship/association, or difference between the study groups or samples. So how can we test to see whether there really is no difference? That's the point we are up to now: the actual test to see whether there is a statistically significant difference.

In this chapter, we are going to talk about the **chi-square (X^2)** test, which is appropriate when you are working with independent samples and an outcome or dependent variable that is nominal- or ordinal-level data. You already know that nominal-level data tells you that there is a difference in the quality of a variable, whereas ordinal level data has a rank order so that one level is greater than or less than another.

For example, suppose you are an operating room nurse and you want to see whether there is a difference between male and female postoperative patients in the need for a postoperative transfusion. Gender the variable that identifies your sample groups. You want to compare a sample of men and a sample of women. Your outcome or dependent variable is postoperative transfusion which is measured at a nominal level (yes/no). Now you want to see whether the frequencies you observe are different from the frequencies you would expect if the variables were independent or not related.

The Null and Alternative Hypotheses

So let's formulate a null and an alternative hypothesis using the standard notation, which looks like this:

H_0: This is how statisticians indicate the null hypothesis.

H_1: This notation indicates the alternative hypothesis.

Here are our hypotheses:

H_0: There is no difference in the need for a postoperative transfusion among men and women.

H_1: The need for a postoperative transfusion is different for men and women.

2 × 2 Table

Your next step is to set up another 2 × 2 table. Statisticians love these! See Figure 8-1.

Figure 8-1 Gender and Postoperative Transfusion Status.

	Male	Female	Total
Transfused	20 (A)	30 (B)	50 (A + B)
Not transfused	30 (C)	20 (D)	50 (C + D)
Total	50 (A + C)	50 (B + D)	100 (A + B + C + D)

Degrees of Freedom

Before you determine statistical significance you will need to determine the **degrees of freedom** (*df*), which is the number values which are "free to be unknown" once the row and column totals are know in a 2 × 2 contingency table. With a chi-square test. the degrees of freedom is equal to the number of rows minus one times the number of columns minus one:

$$df = (2 - 1) \times (2 - 1)$$
$$df = 1 \times 1 = 1$$

All 2 × 2 tables have one degree of freedom. In other words, once you know the row and column totals and one other cell value in the table you can figure out all the rest of the cell values in the table and they do not change unless the original cell value changes. This is why there is only one value which is "free to be unknown."

Statistical Significance

Once you put your data into a statistical program, it will compute the expected values for each of these cells assuming the two variables are independent. You will then need to apply the chi-square test to see whether the observed values are significantly different from the expected values at one degree of freedom.

- If the X^2 result has a *p*-value that is significant (usually < 0.05 depending on the alpha you use), then you reject the null hypothesis that the two variables are independent and conclude that there is an association between gender and postoperative transfusion. Postoperative transfusion rates are significantly different for men and women.
- If the X^2 value is greater than the alpha you selected (i.e., if your alpha is 0.05 and the *p*-value is 0.09), then the result is not statistically significant and you fail to reject the null hypothesis. Your study does not have the statistical strength for you to say the variables are not related. In this case you conclude that post operative transfusion rates are not significantly different for men and women. Remember that this may be because there really isn't a difference in post operative transfusion rates for men and women or because of other reasons, such as your sample size was too small.

Direction of the Relationship

Also note that the chi-square test doesn't tell you the di*rection* of the relationship or difference. If the *p*-value for your X^2 is significant, all you know is that you can reject the null and that there is a statistically significant difference in your outcome variable between the two samples. As the statistical wizard that you are, you then look again at your data to determine what that difference is. For example, if you had a statistically significant X^2 in the example about gender and postoperative transfusions, you could go back and look at which gender had more transfusions. In this sample, a larger portion of the women needed transfusions. Given your statistically significant result, you could conclude that, for this sample, women are more likely to need a postoperative transfusion than men.

FROM THE STATISTICIAN · Brendan Heavey

Pearson's Chi-Square Test for Association

The chi-square test is one of the simplest tests available in a subset of statistics called categorical data analysis. The majority of theories relating to categorical data analysis started to be developed around the turn of the 20th century. Karl Pearson (1857–1936) was a very important statistician from England who is responsible for first developing the chi-squared distribution. Pearson was an arrogant man who frequently butted heads with colleagues. He specifically argued the intelligence and merits of a young statistician named R.A. Fisher (1890–1962), who has since become established as one of the most important scientists of all time. The two men argued over many different things. Fisher was concerned about what would happen to Pearson's chi-squared statistic when sample sizes were extremely low, and Pearson didn't think it was a problem.

Fisher contributed a number of fundamentals of statistical science but specifically in introductory categorical data analysis, he developed the Fisher exact test. This test is now commonly used in place of Pearson's chi-square test when the sample size of any cell in the data is less than 5 (because, in the end, Fisher's arguments with Pearson proved correct). Fisher also used properties derived from Pearson's chi-squared distribution to show that Gregor Mendel, the eminent geneticist and Augustinian priest who theorized about the inheritance of genetic traits using peas, most likely derived many of his theories based on fabricated data. (Fisher remained convinced that one of Mendel's assistants was responsible for the fabrication; Mendel is still considered a very gifted geneticist.) In any event, the two tests—Pearson's chi-square test and Fisher's exact test—are now very common statistics to use in clinical trials and scientific research. Specifically, their use is very popular when a researcher wants to test whether a new treatment or therapy is better than the so-called gold standard already in use.

The null hypothesis that is tested in both these tests is:

H_0: The proportions being compared are equal in the population.

Here is a motivating example, one that's slightly more difficult than the one in the main text. This time we'll use a variable that has more than just two categories!

FROM THE STATISTICIAN   BRENDAN HEAVEY

Suppose we want to study the effect of a husband's occupation on a woman's marital happiness in a clinically relevant population. Our null hypothesis is:

H_0: Husband's occupation has no effect on women's marital happiness in this subset of occupations in the population we've sampled from.

To conduct the study, we enroll 1868 women and ask them to rate the happiness of their marriage on the following four-point scale:

1. Very happy
2. Pretty happy
3. Happy
4. Not too happy

We see the results are shown in Figure 8-2. Now, if you plug these values into any statistical program (or use the FTS methods section from this chapter to hand-calculate the values), you'll see that the p-value for the difference between the happiness of the wives of statisticians versus those of male supermodels is so low that it is estimated at 0. Now you know that there is an association between the husband's occupation and the wife's marital happiness (because your p-value is less than alpha, meaning it is significant). So you reject the null hypothesis that there isn't a relationship between husband's occupation and a wife's marital happiness.

Figure 8-2 Husbands' Occupation and Wives' Report of Marital Happiness.

Marital Happiness	Husbands' Occupation		Total
	Statistician	Male Supermodel	
Very happy	800	25	825
Pretty happy	706	10	716
Happy	200	25	225
Not too happy	2	100	102
Total	1708	160	1868

But what else might you like to know? Let's say that a friend is dating a statistician and a male supermodel and that they both intend to propose this evening. What advice would you give your friend? Which might be the better choice to ensure long-term marital satisfaction? Remember that

(continues)

the chi-square test tells you only that there is a better choice, not which one it is. But you remember from your college stats class that you can determine which is better by looking at the data. The proportion of wives married to statisticians who reported being happy or higher was 99.9% (1706 ÷ 1708), whereas the proportion of wives married to supermodels who reported being happy or higher was 37.5% (60 ÷ 160). So, assuming your friend wants to get married in the first place, which proposal should she accept? (*Hint:* In the statistics books, the statisticians always live happily ever after!)

Here are three health-related studies that all demonstrate the use of this statistic:

1. Corless et al. (2009) examined the effect of marijuana use versus over-the-counter medications for the relief of symptoms and side effects associated with HIV medication.
2. Tobian et al. (2009) investigated the contribution of different variables to determine whether circumcision was an effective strategy for syphilis prevention in a community in Uganda.
3. Anifantaki, S. (2009) examined the relationship between daily interruption of sedative infusions and the duration of mechanical ventilation required in patients in an adult surgical intensive care unit.

[*Note:* All the anecdotal information regarding Spearman and Fisher came from Agresti's (2002) landmark book on the subject, whose name it bears, *Categorical Data Analysis.*]

When *Not* to Use Chi-Square: Assumptions and Special Cases

In a few situations, you might be inclined to use a chi-square test because you have an outcome or dependent variable at the nominal level, but the test wouldn't be a good choice. The chi-square test includes some additional assumptions (in addition to requiring a nominal level outcome or dependent variable), which must be met for the test to be used appropriately.

All cells within the 2 × 2 table must have an observed value greater than or equal to five. If at least one cell in your 2 × 2 table has an observed value < 5 you should use the Fisher exact test instead. You should also note that *if any of the cells in the frequency table have greater than 5 but fewer than 10 expected observations*, you can still use the chi-square test but you need to do a Yates' continuity correction as well. The really nice thing in this day and age is that many statistical programs automatically make this correction when

this condition occurs, saving you the time and trouble of doing it manually. You might want to look for it on your next SPSS printout.

The sample should be random and independent. Here's an example of a violation of this assumption: Your study involved measuring the need for post operative transfusion among husbands and wives who underwent a particular procedure (because these subjects are related to each other they are not independent—once you included the wife in the study the husband was included as well, so his participation was "dependent" on his wife being selected to participate). In this case, the sample is not independent and random. Instead, the sample is now matched, or paired, and a test called the McNemar test is the correct choice to use for the analysis.

(Both the Fisher and the McNemar tests are based on the same idea as the chi-square, but they have mathematical adjustments to accommodate the violation in the assumptions of the chi-square test.)

FROM THE STATISTICIAN   Brendan Heavey

Methods: Calculating Pearson's Chi-Square Test by Hand

Figure 8-3 is a repeat of Figure 8.2 for easier reference.

Figure 8-3 Husbands' Occupation and Wives' Report of Marital Happiness.

	Husbands' Occupation		
Marital Happiness	Statistician	Male Supermodel	Total
Very happy	800	25	825
Pretty happy	706	10	716
Happy	200	25	225
Not too happy	2	100	102
Total	1708	160	1868

1. The first step is to calculate the expected frequency from each cell with the following formula:

$$\text{Expected frequency} = \frac{\text{Row total} \times \text{Column total}}{\text{Grand total}}$$

The results are shown in Figure 8-4.

Figure 8-4 Expected Frequencies for Husbands' Occupation and Wives' Marital Satisfaction.

Expected Frequencies

	Statistician	Male Supermodel
Very happy	(825 × 1708) ÷ 1868 = 754.34	(825 × 160) ÷ 1868 = 70.66
Pretty happy	(716 × 1708) ÷ 1868 = 654.67	(716 × 160) ÷ 1868 = 61.33
Happy	(225 × 1708) ÷ 1868 = 205.73	(225 × 160) ÷ 1868 = 19.27
Not too happy	(102 × 1708) ÷ 1868 = 93.26	(102 × 160) ÷ 1868 = 8.74

(continues)

FROM THE STATISTICIAN	Brendan Heavey

2. Now compute the statistic:

$$\sum \frac{(\text{Observed} - \text{Expected})^2}{\text{Expected}}$$

(The big sigma (Σ) character just means to sum everything over all the cells; in our case we calculate:

$$\frac{(800 - 754.34)^2}{754.37} + \frac{(706 - 654.67)^2}{654.67} + \frac{(200 - 205.73)^2}{205.73} + \frac{(2 - 93.26)^2}{93.26}$$

$$+ \frac{(25 - 70.66)^2}{70.66} + \frac{(10 - 61.33)^2}{61.33} + \frac{(25 - 19.27)^2}{19.27} + \frac{(100 - 8.74)^2}{8.74}$$

Which results in 1123.8.

3. We then apply the formula for calculating the degrees of freedom for a chi-square test:

$$(\text{Number of rows} - 1)(\text{Number of columns} - 1)$$

In this case, the degrees of freedom is:

$$3 \times 1 = 3$$

4. We then look up the p-value for this test statistic from a chi-square distribution with degrees of freedom:

See Appendix C. $p < 0.0001$.

Summary

There are two main points to review in this chapter.

First, you should have the concept of the null hypothesis in your head by now from seeing it in almost every chapter! The null hypothesis is that there is no relationship/association, or difference between the variables of interest. If you are still having trouble with it, we will visit it again.

Second, the chi-square test is used to look for a statistically significant difference or relationship when you have a nominal- or ordinal-level dependent or outcome variable.

- If the chi-square test result has a p-value that is significant (less than 0.05 or whatever alpha you use), then you reject the null hypothesis.
- If the chi-square test result is not statistically significant (greater than 0.05 or the alpha of choice), then you fail to reject the null hypothesis.

The chi-square test does not tell you the direction of the relationship; only you can make that interpretation.

That about wraps up this chapter. Not too bad, right?!

CHAPTER 8 REVIEW QUESTIONS

Questions 1–11: A study is completed to examine the relationship between gender and sports participation. It is conducted by randomly surveying ninth-graders at Smith High School. The collected data is shown in Figure 8-5.

Figure 8-5 Gender and Sports Participation Among Ninth-Grade Students.

	Male	Female	Total
No sports	30	50	80
Sports participation	70	50	120
Total	100	100	200

1. What level of measurement is gender? Is it continuous or categorical?

2. What level of measurement is sports participation? Is it qualitative or quantitative?

3. What measure of central tendency can you determine for sports participation? What is the measure of central tendency for males only? Is the measure of central tendency different for the whole sample?

4. If the whole school has 800 students and the ninth grade has 250 students, what percentage of the ninth-grade population did you sample?

(continues)

5. Write an appropriate null hypothesis for this study.

_____

_____

6. Write two alternative hypotheses that correspond to your null hypothesis.

   (1) _____

   _____

   (2) _____

   _____

7. Calculate the chi-square from the 2 × 2 table in Figure 8-5. The p-value is < 0.005. Is sports participation significantly different for males and females in this sample? (See the FTS Methods calculation.)

_____

_____

8. What you should conclude about your null hypothesis?

_____

_____

9. What type of error might you be making?

_____

10. If you wanted to make the chance of this type of error smaller, what could you do?

_____

11. Why is the chi-square test appropriate for this study?

_____

Questions 12–14: After the school instituted a new aerobics program, data was gathered in a follow-up survey administered in all the grades. The collected information is shown in Figure 8-6.

12. If the entire school has a population of 800, what percentage of the students are included in your sample?

_____

Figure 8-6 Gender and Sports Participation After New Aerobics Program.

	Male	Female	Total
No sports	60	20	80
Sports participation	140	180	320
Total	200	200	400

Chi-square $= 25, p < 0.0001$

13. Is gender related to sport participation in this follow-up survey? If so, which gender is more likely to participate? How many degrees of freedom do you have?

_____

_____

_____

14. Imagine you are the editor of the journal in which an article was submitted for review using a chi-square test to determine if boys or girls were more likely to participate in sports. After reading it, you realize that the male and female subjects were recruited as brother and sister pairs. What would you conclude about the analysis?

_____

15. You are working in a school-based health center and have developed a new screening tool for suicide risk among adolescent athletes. The pilot of your new screening tool reports female athletes are more likely to attempt suicide when compared to male athletes. These results agree with other published reports from the general adolescent population. This helps establish what type of validity for your new screen?

_____

16. You administer your new screen in your health clinic but find the results confusing. After reviewing your tool, you realize that a mistake was made. When the survey was administered to three of the male sports teams, it was printed on only one side of the paper and should have been copied onto both sides. As a result, half of the survey was missing when it was administered to these three teams. Is your screen reliable? What does this tell you about the validity of the screen in this situation?

_____

_____

(continues)

17. You correct the copying problem and readminister the screen at another school. After one year of follow-up, you get the results shown in Figure 8-7. Explain what each box means in English.

_____

_____

_____

_____

Figure 8-7 Suicide Risk and Screening Results.

	Attempt Suicide	No Suicide Attempt	Total
Screen positive	20	5	25
Screen negative	10	215	225
Total	30	220	250

18. What is the sensitivity of your screen? What does this mean in English?

_____

19. What is the specificity of your screen? What does this mean in English?

_____

20. What is the PPV of your screen? What does this mean in English?

_____

21. What is the NPV of your screen? What does this mean in English?

_____

22. What is the prevalence of suicide attempts in this sample?

_____

FTS REVIEW QUESTION

23. Would you do the analysis differently if no women were happily married to male supermodels in the FTS in this chapter?

_____

_____

_____

Use your computer to practice these applications.

The companion website for this book has a computer-based application example for this material. Check it out!

| Analyze | Graphs | Utilities | Add-ons | Window | Help |

Reports ▶

Descriptive Statistics ▶

Tables ▶

Compare Means ▶

General Linear Model ▶

Generalized Linear Models ▶

Frequencies...

Descriptives...

Explore...

Crosstabs...

ANSWERS TO CHAPTER 8 REVIEW QUESTIONS

1. Nominal, categorical

3. Nominal, mode, mode = participating in sports for males and for the total sample

5. H_0: There is no relationship between gender and sports participation

7.

$$\sum \frac{(\text{Observed} - \text{Expected})^2}{\text{Expected}}$$

$$\frac{(30 - 40)^2}{40} + \frac{(50 - 40)^2}{40} + \frac{(70 - 60)^2}{60} + \frac{(50 - 60)^2}{60}$$

$$= 100/40 + 100/40 + 100/60 + 100/60 = 8.34$$

$$df = 1$$

See Figure 8-8.

Figure 8-8 Expected Values for Gender and Sports Participation.

	Male	Female
No sports	$(80 \times 100) \div 200 = 40$	$(80 \times 100) \div 200 = 40$
Sports participation	$(120 \times 100) \div 200 = 60$	$(120 \times 100) \div 200 = 60$

If your alpha is 0.05 then yes sports participation is significantly different for males and females. This conclusion is because p is significant.

9. Type one

11. The outcome variable is nominal/ordinal, it is an independent sample and the cell values are all > 5.

13. Yes, females are more likely.

$$df = (\text{Number of rows} - 1) \times (\text{Number of columns} - 1) = 1 \times 1 = 1$$

15. Convergent

17. 20 = true positives, 5 = false positives, 10 = false negatives, 215 = true negatives

19. 215/220 = 98%. If the subject does not have the disease there is a 98% chance the screen will be negative. A specific screen is good at identifying those without the disease.

21. 215/225 = 96%. If the screening test is negative, it is the probability that the subject does not have the disease.

ANSWER TO CHAPTER 8 FTS QUESTION

23. You would need to use Fisher's exact test because of the small cell size.

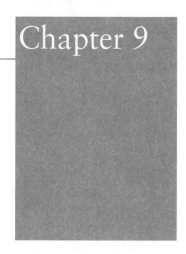

Chapter 9

Student *t*-Test

How can I find a difference in the two sample means if my dependent variable is at the interval or ratio level?

OBJECTIVES

By the end of the chapter students will be able to:

- Identify the conditions under which the student *t*-test is an appropriate statistical technique.

- Compare and contrast dependent and independent samples.

- Identify independent and dependent samples in current nursing research.

- Write null and alternative hypotheses that demonstrate an understanding of student *t*-test.

- Calculate the degrees of freedom associated with a given data set.

- Interpret the SPSS output from a student *t*-test, and determine whether it is statistically significant; interpret this result in statistical terms and in plain English; prepare a public health report using the information.

- Critique an article from current nursing research that utilizes a student *t*-test; determine what type of sample was collected; identify whether the samples were independent or dependent; determine whether statistical significance is present, and debate whether clinical recommendations should be made.

KEY TERMS

Degrees of freedom for t-tests
Equals the sample size for both groups minus two.

Dependent samples
Paired or related groups or the same sample at a different time.

Independent samples
Do not have a relationship with each other.

Noninferiority trial
A trial used to show that a new treatment is no worse than an old procedure (may use a one-tailed test).

Sampling error
Error that occurs due to randomization and chance.

Student t-test
Used when you are looking for a difference in the mean value of an interval or ratio level variable.

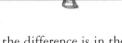

The Student *t*-Test

One of our favorite statistical tests is called a student *t*-test, which was developed by William Gossett.

Appropriate Use of the Student *t*-Test

Before you can apply the student *t*-test to determine whether there is a difference between the means in the two sample groups, you need to determine three things:

- What is the level of measurement for the outcome variable?
- Are there two samples?
- Are the samples independent?

Level of Measurement

The student *t*-test is appropriate only when you are looking for a difference in the mean value of an outcome variable that is at the interval or ratio level. In this case, the difference is in the amount of epinephrine in the injectors, which is a ratio level measurement (i.e., it shows a difference with equal ranked intervals and has a zero value); so it is appropriate.

The next question is what kind of samples do you have? First of all, are there two samples? To look for a difference in the mean value of the outcome variable, you must have at least two samples. In the injector example, you have a sample of injectors from Acme and a sample of injectors from EPI. So you have two samples, and you are looking for a difference in the mean amount of epinephrine found in each.

Now that you know you have two samples, you have to ask did how you selected one sample affect the other? In the example, the two samples were randomly collected from two different kinds of injectors without any relationship to each other; so these are two **independent samples**. However, suppose you collected one sample of Acme injectors, measured their mean epinephrine levels pre-administration, gave the injections, and

FROM THE STATISTICIAN   Brendan Heavey

Let's Talk t-Tests

Fueled by the success of scrubs sales by Carol's Nursing Scrubs, Carol has decided to expand her product offering to include injectable epinephrine pens. Carol has asked you to decide which type of pen she should retail. Two production companies are competing for the job: Acme Pens and EphedraPens International (EPI). They both produce injections that are advertised to hold 0.3 mg of epinephrine. The snag is that both companies have had some bad press recently over the amount of epinephrine in their products. Carol has asked you to check up on each company and decide whether one type of pen holds more epinephrine than the other.

In this scenario, you're interested in comparing the average amount of epinephrine in Acme's pens with the average amount of epinephrine in EPI's pens—two population parameters. The two companies are not going to give you access to their production facility to test out the whole population of pens. So you need to take a sample of each and make some inferences. Obviously, the samples from separate companies are independent of each other.

If it weren't for a man named William Gosset (1876–1937), answering questions like this would be much more difficult. After completing a degree at Oxford in 1899, Gosset decided to do what many other great Celtic men in history did and went to work for the Guinness brewery in Dublin, Ireland. While there, he was enlisted to work on projects to help decide how the quality of hops and barley affected the taste of a "pint 'o the black stuff" (the proper way to refer to a glass of Guinness beer in Dublin). After Guinness sent him to study under a great statistician by the name of Karl Pearson, Gosset published a landmark paper that derived the *t*-distribution in 1908. Guinness considered his work top secret, and, as a result, he was forced to publish under the pen name "Student." This is why the *t*-distribution is sometimes referred to as "Student's *t*" or **student *t*-test**, which is used when you are looking for a difference in the mean value of an interval- or ratio-level variable.

Due to Gosset's work, we know we can perform an independent samples *t*-test on our epinephrine injection data to determine whether there is a statistical difference between the amounts of epinephrine in the two overall populations of injectors.

Note: All factual information regarding William Gossett was taken from Johnson & Kotz (1997).

then measured the residual epinephrine levels post-administration to see if there was a difference. (Obviously, if you are injecting the epinephrine there should be!) In that case, you would still have two samples, but they would be **dependent**, or related. Your second sample is a remeasurement of the same sample group at a different point in time.

You can also have dependent samples when you match sample characteristics. For example,

if you are interested in comparing the average duration of hospital stay for individuals at two different hospitals, you might decide you want both samples to have been admitted for the same diagnosis. So you randomly sample 10 patients at the first hospital and measure their length of stay. Then you go to the second hospital and randomly select 10 subjects with the same admission diagnosis as the first group. Because those selected for your second sample have to have had the same diagnosis as your first sample, they are not independent samples; they are correlated, or dependent. You can still determine whether the average length of stay differed depending on the hospital by comparing the mean from each group. However, to do this accurately, you have to use a *t*-test for dependent groups because that is the type of sample you have.

However, in the epinephrine injectors example, you know you have an outcome variable that is at the ratio level and two samples that are independent and randomly collected. The presence of these factors means that you can apply the student *t*-test for independent groups. (Two other factors—normal distribution of the outcome variable and homogeneity of variance—are ideally also present, but they are not absolutely essential, even though they do impact statistical interpretation. You can explore these factors more fully in the upcoming FTS section!)

So, before applying an independent student *t*-test, simply answer the following questions:

- Is my outcome variable at the interval or ratio level?
- Do I have two samples?
- Are my samples random and independent from one another?

If your answers to these three questions are yes, you may proceed with a student *t*-test for independent groups.

The Null and Alternative Hypotheses

In the example, the null hypothesis is that there is no difference between the mean amounts of epinephrine in the two types of Epinephrine injectors. Our alternative hypothesis, therefore,

is that there is a difference between the mean amounts of epinephrine in the two types of pens. We collect our first sample of pens from Acme and find that the average amount of epinephrine in each injector is 0.31 mg. We then collect our second sample of pens from EPI and find the average amount is 0.30 mg. There is a difference in the sample means, but is it statistically significant or is it just due to **sampling error** (error that occurs due to randomization and chance)? Because this appears to be a relatively small difference between the means, it is unlikely to be significant, but remember that it could be if the sample size is large.

Statistical Significance

To determine whether the difference is statistically significant, you have to decide on a number of things:

- *The level of risk you are going to take that you will incorrectly reject the null hypothesis (alpha):* For this example, you decide to take a 5% chance that you will make a type one error. So you select an alpha of 0.05.
- *The power (the chance of finding a difference if it actually exists):* You decide that 0.80, or 80%, is adequate.
- *Whether you are conducting a one-tailed or two-tailed test:* These terms simply indicate whether you are looking for a difference in either direction (two-tailed) or you have you hypothesized that the difference is in a specific direction such as the mean in the second sample is greater than or less than the mean in the first (one-tailed)? Because this example is looking for a difference in any direction between the epinephrine levels in the two groups, you are going to do a two-tailed student *t*-test.

FROM THE STATISTICIAN   BRENDAN HEAVEY

Using a One-Tailed Test

Using one-sided, or one-tailed, hypothesis test is a controversial procedure that should be avoided in most instances. The researcher who is interested in a *directional* null hypothesis would use a one-tailed test. The assumption is that, based on prior information or previous testing, there is no chance of a change in one of the two possible directions for a particular variable. Therefore, alpha (α), which is usually split between two tails, has its probability shifted to one tail (or one side), as we see in Figure 9-1.

One-tailed tests are sometimes acceptable. Their most common use is in **noninferiority trials**, whose point is to show that a new treatment is no worse than an old procedure. For example, a new noninvasive procedure is found that might be a replacement for an older invasive procedure. We don't want to show that the new procedure is better than the old one, only that it is no worse. In this case, using a one-tailed test makes sense because the probability in the *upper* or right side of the tail would indicate that our new noninvasive procedure performed better than our old procedure. Because there is virtually no likelihood of this occurring, we shift the probability to the *lower* or left side of the tail. In this case, we are testing the following null and alternative hypotheses:

H_0: There is no difference between the two therapies
H_1: The change in response from one therapy is *less than* the change in response from another.

If we were using a two-tailed test, the alternative hypothesis would like this:

H_1: The change in response from one therapy is *different from* the change in response from another.

Can you see the difference between these two alternative hypotheses?

Some researchers overuse one-tailed tests. Why is this practice a problem? Can you figure out why we cannot use one-tailed tests all the time? Is it easier or more difficult to attain statistical significance with a one-tailed test? Let's look at a scenario in which a one-sided test is inappropriate.

Let's say you are working for a pharmaceutical company that has discovered a new drug to treat the flu. The drug is suspected to reduce fever; so your company has you test this hypothesis with the following procedure:

- Enroll 200 subjects who have the flu.
- Administer the test drug to 100 subjects and a placebo sugar pill to the other 100.
- Wait 4 hours and then take everyone's temperature.

In this case, let's say we use a two-sample student *t*-test to test the difference between average temperatures in these two groups four hours after they take the test or placebo pill. You end up with data as shown in Figure 9-2.

The corresponding *p*-value is not significant when we use a two-tailed test, but it is if we use a one-tailed test.

(continues)

FROM THE STATISTICIAN   Brendan Heavey

If you're working for the drug company that is pressing to get this new drug to market, you might use a one-sided test based on the argument that there is no chance the new drug will increase fever. Switching to a one-sided test would be a violation of a number of issues: You did not decide which test you were going to use beforehand, and you have no prior research to suggest that the pill could not elevate a fever. Needless to say, using a one-tailed test in this situation is not advisable. In fact, one-tailed testing is so frowned upon that some scientific journals require only two-sided *p*-values to be reported. This policy is in place to prevent researchers from cheating and attaining statistical significance in their work too easily.

For examples of appropriate one-sided tests in the literature, see:

- *The Diamond trial:* A non-invasive ultrasound procedure was tested against amniocentesis, an older and more invasive procedure to test for severe fetal anemia. (Oepkes, 2006).
- *Neuroblastoma screening:* Researchers investigated whether neuroblastoma screening in infancy improved the survival of children diagnosed with this disease (Schilling, 2002).
- *Effect of lidocaine during breast biopsy:* Researchers determined that applying topical lidocaine decreased the pain women experienced during breast biopsy (Olbrys, 2001).

Figure 9-1 Location of Alpha (α) with a Two-Sided Versus One-Sided Test.

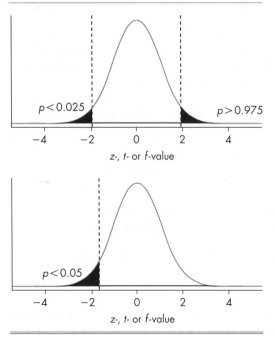

Figure 9-2 Clinical Trial for New Flu Medication.

	Average Temperature After
Drug	101.2
Placebo	102.1

Degrees of Freedom for Student *t*-Tests

This test involves one other concept: **degrees of freedom**, which is equal to the sample size for both groups minus two. This is the same as taking the degrees of freedom for each group (sample size for the group minus one) and adding them together. Now you might feel as though you have no freedom, but in your study you do; let's see how much. When you collect a sample of 10 injectors and measure their epinephrine levels, you have 10 values that are "free" to vary depending on which injectors you select and how much epinephrine is in each. However, once you calculate the mean level of epinephrine, only 9 of the values are actually free to be "unknown" at any one time. Once you know the amount of epinephrine in each of the nine injector pens and you know the mean, you can figure out how much epinephrine is in the last injector. The value for the last injector pen is no longer free to vary; so when you calculate the mean, you lose a degree of freedom.

If degrees of freedom still has you totally baffled, just remember this: Take your total sample size (both groups) minus two (one from each group), and you know the degrees of freedom for the test (see Figure 9-3). Then all you need to do is find the right location on the table (see Appendix C of the book).

(You can still perform a student *t*-test without really understanding this concept! Just don't tell the statisticians I said so!)

So when are we getting to the really exciting student *t*-test? The *t*-test equation appears in any basic statistics textbook—except this one. The reality of nursing work today is that you won't be making the calculation. Sorry! Okay, for those of you who really want to see the equation, you can check it out in the next FTS Methods. All the rest of you need only to be able to look at a computer printout or a research article and understand what it means.

Figure 9-3 Formula for Calculating Degrees of Freedom for Student *t*-Tests.

$$\text{Degrees of freedom} = (n_1 + n_2) - 2$$

where
n_1 = total number of subjects in sample one
n_2 = total number of subjects in sample two

FROM THE STATISTICIAN   BRENDAN HEAVEY

Methods: Student's t-Test

Student's *t*-test is so named because it makes use of what is called the *t*-statistical distribution. The test is probably the most often used statistical test, for better or worse. I say "for better or worse" because it's not always the correct test to run; it's just usually the most straightforward.

The purpose of a two-sample *t*-test is to determine whether the means of two groups differ significantly.

The *t*-test has a few versions; so you have to ask a few questions before performing one:

1. *How many tails (one or two) of the statistical distribution do you want to test?* (For an in-depth discussion of this topic, see the FTS "Using a One-Tailed Test" earlier in the chapter.)
2. *Is your data paired?* In some instances, data is set up so that the two groups under consideration have members that are paired instead of being independent. An example of paired data occurs in a so-called crossover clinical trial, in which subjects are given both a placebo and a drug (as shown in Figure 9-4). Setting up a trial in this manner is suitable for a paired analysis because each subject has two measures taken: one with the placebo and one with the drug. Because these measures are not measured on two different subjects, the *t*-test that compares their outcomes must be adjusted to account for their non-independence and a repeated measures test for the different in dependent samples should be used.

(continues)

FROM THE STATISTICIAN   BRENDAN HEAVEY

3. *Can you assume equal variances in the two different groups?* One of the assumptions of the two-sample *t*-test is that the two groups have the same variance. Slight departures from this assumption are okay, but if they are too extreme, a different formula should be used. (That alternative is beyond the scope of this book.) Statisticians describe this property as homogeneity of variance or equal variances. (You can try out that vocabulary at your next racquetball match!)

Here's an example of an independent-sample *t*-test to determine if there is a difference in the mean age between two mutually exclusive groups. Data was collected on trauma cases aged 25 and under during one 72-hour period at an upstate New York tertiary care facility. We were interested in comparing the mean ages between groups who did have a positive drug screen and those who did not. The data set used is shown in Figure 9-5. We ran a basic analysis in SPSS, whose output is shown in Figures 9-6 through 9-10.

Is the homogeneity of variance assumption appropriate to use in this case? Let's look at the standard deviations of the two groups. We see that the drug-screen-negative group has a standard deviation of 8.54593, whereas the drug-screen-positive group has a standard deviation of 3.28634 (Figure 9-9). Tests are available that can be used to decide whether the equivariance assumption holds. The SPSS we chose used Levene's test for equality of variances. Note the large discrepancy in the standard deviations compared to their overall magnitude, and agree that they are pretty far off from each other. Levene's test for equality of variances tests the null hypothesis that the variances in the two groups are not different. In this example, the Levene's test for equality of variances has a significant *p*-value so you reject the null hypothesis that the variances are equal and use the second line of the *t*-test analysis (for when equal variances are not assumed). That line shows a *t*-value of -1.294, which converts to a two-tailed *p*-value of 0.212. Since the study had an alpha of 0.05, you know that this *p*-value is not adequate to reject H_0. Therefore, you fail to reject H_0: There is not enough evidence to suggest there is a difference in the mean ages of patients in the two groups of a positive and a negative drug screen.

Let's look at a brief computation that explains what makes up the *t*-value. If the standard deviations for the two groups were similar and we therefore assumed equal variances, you would calculate the appropriate *t*-value (T) by means of the following formula:

$$T = \frac{\bar{X}_1 - \bar{X}_2}{SE}$$

The difference between the means ($\bar{X}_1 - \bar{X}_2$) was -3.42857, and the standard error (SE) of the difference, assuming equal variances, was 3.64319; so the calculation looks like this:

$$\frac{-3.42857}{3.64319} = -0.941$$

Notice that -0.941 is the *t*-value associated with the test on the statistical computing output table (Figure 9-10). If you did not assume equal variances, the denominator would be the standard error of the difference of 2.64, and the resulting *t*-value would be -1.294 (see Figure 9-10).

Figure 9-4 Cross-Over Study Design.

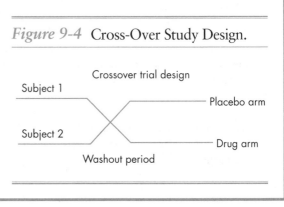

Figure 9-5 Age and Drug Screen Status for Patients Under Age 25 in a Trauma Center.

Age	Drug Screen	Age	Drug Screen
2	0	20	0
3	0	20	1
5	0	20	1
7	0	21	1
8	0	22	0
15	1	22	0
15	1	23	1
18	0	23	0
19	0	25	0
19	0	25	0

Drug screen: 0 = negative, 1 = positive

Figure 9-6 Frequency Table for Age.

		Age		
	Frequency	Percentage	Valid Percentage	Cumulative Percentage
Valid 2	1	5.0	5.0	5.0
3	1	5.0	5.0	10.0
5	1	5.0	5.0	15.0
7	1	5.0	5.0	20.0
8	1	5.0	5.0	25.0
15	2	10.0	10.0	35.0
18	1	5.0	5.0	40.0
19	2	10.0	10.0	50.0
20	3	15.0	15.0	65.0
21	1	5.0	5.0	70.0
22	2	10.0	10.0	80.0
23	2	10.0	10.0	90.0
25	2	10.0	10.0	100.0
Total	20	100.0	100.0	

Figure 9-7 Descriptive Statistics for Age Variable.

Statistics

Age

N	Valid	20.0000
	Missing	0.0000
Mean		16.6000
Median		19.5000
Mode		20.0000
Standard deviation		7.4438
Variance		55.4105
Skewness		−0.9158
Standard error of skewness		0.5121
Percentiles	25	9.7500
	50	19.5000
	75	22.0000

Figure 9-8 Bar Chart for Age Variable.

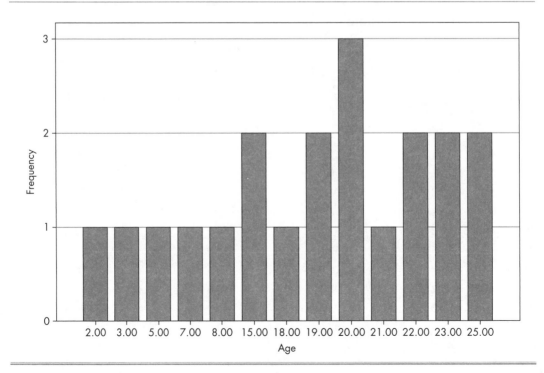

Figure 9-9 Means by Drug Screen Status.

Group Statistics

Drug Screen		N	Mean	Standard Deviation	Standard Error Mean
Age	Negative	14	15.5714	8.54593	2.28400
	Positive	6	19.0000	3.28634	1.34164

Figure 9-10 *t*-Test for Equality of Mean Age Between Those with a Negative and Those with a Positive Drug Screen.

Independent Samples Test

		Levene's Test for Equality of Variances		t-Test for Equality of Means						
									95% Confidence Interval of the Difference	
		F	Significance	t	df	Significance (2-tailed)	Mean Difference	Standard Error Difference	Lower	Upper
Age	Equal variances assumed	11.098	0.004	−0.941	18	0.359	−3.42857	3.64319	−11.08264	4.22550
	Equal variances not assumed			−1.294	17.960	0.212	−3.42857	2.64889	−8.99459	2.13745

Summary

You have just completed Chapter 9. Very impressive! Now let's review the main points.

First and foremost, remember that the null hypothesis is that there is no difference between the group means. The student *t*-test is used to determine whether there is a difference in an interval- or ratio-level outcome or dependent variable in two sample groups. If the sample groups are independent, the sample groups do not have any relationship. If the samples are dependent, the groups are matched on an attribute or may be the same group measured at a different time, in either case they are related to each other. The sampling error occurs due to randomization or chance, and the degrees of freedom equals the total sample size minus two.

If you had difficulty with the chapter, review it several more times because you want to assimilate these concepts well before learning newer and more difficult concepts. When you are confident in your knowledge of this material, move on!

CHAPTER 9 REVIEW QUESTIONS

Questions 1–11: You are asked to design a study determining whether there is a difference in the average fasting blood glucose for individuals with diabetes randomized either to a strictly dietary intervention or to a diet and exercise intervention.

1. Are you looking for a relationship/association or a difference?

   _____

2. What is your dependent variable?

   _____

3. Is it qualitative or quantitative? Is it continuous or categorical? What level of measurement is it?

   _____

   _____

   _____

4. How many samples do you have? Is this a probability or nonprobability sampling method?

   _____

   _____

5. Are these independent or dependent groups?

_____

6. Would you prefer to use a chi-square test or a student *t*-test with this study?

_____

7. Write appropriate null and alternative hypotheses.

Null: _____

_____

_____

Alternative: _____

_____

8. Your study includes an alpha of 0.05 and a power of 0.80. You conduct a student *t*-test, which has a *p*-value of 0.07. What is your conclusion?

_____

_____

9. What type of error might you be making?

_____

10. A trial is repeated with a larger sample and the student *t*-test has a *p*-value of 0.04. What is your conclusion now?

_____

_____

11. What type of error might you be making now?

_____

Questions 12–24: Chung and Hwang (2008) examined the difference between an experimental and control group of patients with leukemia. The experimental group received two follow-up phone calls after discharge, and the control group received routine care. Their Table 2 is reproduced as Figure 9-11.

(continues)

12. What was the independent variable?

13. What were the dependent variables?

14. What was the mean score for the quality of life for each group?

15. Which group had a higher quality of life 4 weeks after discharge? Was this statistically significant?

16. What was the mean score for self-care for each group?

17. Which group had the ability to provide more of its own self-care? Was this a statistically significant difference?

18. Which group had a higher level of symptom distress? Was this statistically significant?

19. Interpret these findings in English, and give a plausible explanation for them.

20. Look at Figure 9-12 from the same study. Interpret the statistically significant results in English.

21. Did the experimental group have higher levels of any symptom of distress?

_____

22. A convenience sample was used. Is this a probability or non-probability sampling method?

_____

23. How might this affect the results?

_____

24. How could you improve on this study's sampling method?

_____

Questions 25–31: You are conducting a small study at your hospital looking at infants born in the first 24 hours after the conclusion of a hurricane. You classify prematurity status as full-term (0) if the infants are born after 37 weeks of gestation and premature (1) if they are born before 37 weeks gestation. You measure birth weight in grams at the time of delivery. You conduct a *t*-test to see whether the mean birth weights differ between the premature and full term infants. See Figures 9-13 and 9-14.

25. What is your sample size?

_____

26. What is the mean birth weight for full-term infants?

_____

27. What is the mean birth weight for preterm infants?

_____

28. Which group has a larger standard deviation?

_____

29. Since the Levene's test for equality of variances is not significant, the standard practice is to assume equal variances. What is the appropriate *t*-value?

_____

30. Is the *t*-value significant?

_____

31. What do you conclude?

_____

Figure 9-11 Test of Two-Group Differences 4 Weeks After Discharge.

Variable	Experimental Group (N = 35)		Control Group (N = 35)		
	X	SD	X	SD	t
Self-care	2.67	0.36	1.78	0.38	10.347*
Symptom distress	0.34	0.21	0.82	0.51	−5.158*
Quality of life	70.46	18.76	44.15	16.01	6.074*

*$p < 0.001$

Source: From Chung & Hwang (2008). Copyright 2008 by the Oncology Nursing Society. Reprinted and translated with permission. ONS assumes no responsibility for the accuracy or quality of the translation..

Figure 9-12 Test of Two-Group Differences of Symptom Distress.

Variable	Experimental Group (N = 35)		Control Group (N = 35)		
	X	SD	X	SD	t
Appetite change	1.00	1.59	1.66	1.24	−1.931
Fatigue	1.00	0.59	2.11	1.13	−5.158***
Appearance change	1.14	1.03	1.54	1.15	−1.533
Nausea	0.43	0.61	0.46	0.74	0.464
Irritability	0.29	0.46	0.86	0.73	−3.909***
Change in sexual interest	0.71	0.83	1.23	1.17	−2.131
Insomnia (sleeplessness)	0.17	0.38	1.09	1.20	−4.303***
Dry mouth	0.34	0.48	1.23	1.06	−4.502***
Pain	0.37	0.65	0.97	1.22	−2.564
Dizziness	0.43	0.65	0.51	0.78	−0.498
Lack of concentration	0.23	0.43	0.94	0.87	−4.325***
Numbness	0.26	0.44	0.83	0.79	−3.748***
Diarrhea	—	—	0.29	0.52	−3.260**
Chest discomfort	0.09	0.37	0.43	0.70	−2.562*
Oral or esophageal ulcer	0.26	0.44	0.49	0.89	−1.364
Stomach discomfort	0.09	0.28	0.23	0.49	−1.492
Dyspnea	0.11	0.40	1.02	3.57	−1.506
Bleeding	0.11	0.40	0.49	0.92	−2.188*
Cough	0.17	0.38	0.60	0.81	−2.826**
Trembling	0.09	0.37	0.43	0.74	−2.449*
Fever	0.06	0.24	0.40	0.74	−2.626*
Dysuria	0.09	0.37	0.14	0.69	−0.430

*$p < 0.05$; **$p < 0.01$; *** $p < 0.001$

Source: From Chung & Hwang (2008). Copyright 2008 by the Oncology Nursing Society. Reprinted and translated with permission. ONS assumes no responsibility for the accuracy or quality of the translation.

Figure 9-13 Mean Birth Weight for Full-Term and Premature Infants.

Group Statistics

Preterm Status		I	Mean	Standard. Deviation	Standard Error Mean
Birth weight	0	6	3453.3333	435.41551	177.75764
	1	4	1225.0000	357.07142	178.53571

Figure 9-14 *t*-Test for Equality of Mean Birth Weight in Full-Term and Premature Infants.

Independent Samples Test

		Levene's Test for Equality of Variances		*t*-Test for Equality of Means					95% Confidence Interval of the Difference	
		F	Significance	*t*	df	Significance (2-tailed)	Mean Difference	Standard Error Difference	Lower	Upper
Birth weight	Equal variances assumed	0.767	0.407	8.465	8	0.000	2228.33333	263.23640	1621.30910	2835.35756
	Equal variances not assumed			7.484		0.000	2228.33333	251.93804	1640.30927	2816.35740

CHAPTER 9 FTS REVIEW QUESTION

32. The appropriate *t*-value when not assuming equal variances has been removed from the table in Figure 9.14. Calculate what it would be.

Use your computer to practice these applications.
The companion website for this book has a computer-based application example for this material. Check it out!

ANSWERS TO CHAPTER 9 REVIEW QUESTIONS

1. Difference

3. Quantitative, continuous, interval/ratio

5. Independent

7. Answers may vary, for example:

   H_0: There is no difference in fasting blood glucose in the diet-only group versus the diet and exercise group.

   H_1: There is a difference in the fasting blood glucose for the two groups.

9. Type II

11. Type one

13. Self-care, symptom distress, quality of life

15. Experimental, yes

17. Experimental, yes

19. Telephone support worked, or the experimental group was just healthier. (They had lower signs and symptoms of distress, and there was nonrandom assignment and no pretest; so we don't know whether this group was just healthier to start with.)

21. No

23. The groups may have been significantly different before the intervention.

25. 10

27. 1225 g

29. 8.465

31. Reject the null. There is a significant difference in the mean age of premature infants and full-term infants in this sample

Analysis of Variance (ANOVA)

How do I compare the dependent variable means from more than two samples?

OBJECTIVES

By the end of the chapter students will be able to:

- Describe the conditions in which ANOVA would be an appropriate test.

- Write null and alternative hypotheses that demonstrate understanding of the guiding principles of ANOVA.

- Determine whether ANOVA test results are significant.

- Describe ANOVA study results in plain English.

- Compare ANOVA and repeat-measures ANOVA.

- Relate situations in which repeat-measures ANOVA would be useful and why.

- Express some limitations or concerns associated with repeat-measures ANOVA.

- Critique a current nursing research article that uses ANOVA and interpret the results statistically and in plain English; prepare a public health report using this information.

KEY TERMS

ANOVA (analysis of variance)
The test used when comparing the means from a single dependent variable among two or more groups or samples.

Carry-over effects
Occur when previous treatments continue to have an effect through the next treatment, affecting the measurement of the dependent variable.

Compound symmetry
Measurements are correlated and of equal variances.

Homogeneity of variance
Equal variances among the groups being compared.

Position or latency effects
Occur when a subject is being exposed to more than one treatment over time and the order of the treatment received impacts the outcome.

Power
Probability of detecting a difference that really exists.

Repeat-measures ANOVA
Examines a change over time in the same sample population.

Comparing More Than Two Samples

So far we've talked about how to find a difference between two groups when you have an outcome variable that is a nominal or ordinal level of measurement (chi-square test) and if you have an outcome variable that is a interval or ratio level of measurement (*t*-test). But all that discussion assumed examining the differences between only two independent samples. What if you have more than two samples or groups? You could do multiple *t*-tests, but you could do only two groups at a time, and each comparison would have a risk of a type one error equal to alpha (e.g., 0.05). Even doing three *t*-tests to compare three groups (1 + 2, 2 + 3, 1 + 3) increases the risk of a type one error to 0.05 + 0.05 + 0.05, or 0.15, which is substantial. For this reason, statisticians prefer to use a different test called **analysis of variance (ANOVA)** when comparing more than two group or sample means.

The Null and Alternative Hypotheses

Suppose you are working on a study to examine the average systolic blood pressure of men from different racial groups. Your sample includes subjects who are Caucasian (group 1), African-American (group 2), and Latino (group 3). Your null hypothesis is that all the men will have a similar mean systolic blood pressure regardless of racial background.

$$H_0: M_1 = M_2 = M_3$$

The alternative hypothesis is:

$$H_1: \text{The three means are not equal.}$$

(Note: They don't all have to be unequal. Even if two are significantly unequal, you would reject the null hypothesis.)

The analysis of variance test determines whether the differences seen in the sample means are significantly larger than one would expect by mere chance. An equation then produces an *F*-ratio that relates the differences between the groups (the numerator) to the difference within the groups (the denominator). (For those of you who are interested check out the FTS Methods box at the end of the chapter- You can study the equation to your heart's content.)

When the null hypothesis is correct and there isn't a difference in the means of the groups being studied, the *F*-ratio is close to one. In that case, the differences between the groups are very similar to the differences within the groups (due to normal individual differences), and the *F*-ratio is not significant.

Degrees of Freedom

As usual, there is also a measure of degrees of freedom. The difference is that the numerator of the *F*-ratio has one number for degrees of freedom (number of groups minus one) and the denominator of the *F*-ratio has another (the number of subjects minus the number of groups). When you add the two, the sum becomes the degrees of freedom associated with the *F*-ratio.

Statistical Significance

The *F*-ratio is like any other statistical measure in that it has a *p*-value that determines its significance. You can look up the *p*-value on a table for the *F*-distribution, or you can just program your statistical computing package to tell you what it is. (Personally, I much prefer when my computer does the work but the *F*-distribution tables are in Appendix C if you would like to check them out yourself.) If the *p*-value is less than the alpha you select (i.e., 0.05), then you have the statistical strength to reject the null hypothesis and report that there is a difference among the average blood pressures of the three

samples or groups. If, on the other hand, you have an alpha of 0.05 and your *F*-ratio has a *p*-value of 0.09, you must fail to reject the null and conclude that you do not have the statistical power to show a difference or that there really isn't one.

In your study of systolic blood pressure in men from different racial groups, let's say you find that the average for group 1 is 142, group 2's is 145, and group 3's is 128. Your *F*-ratio has a *p*-value of 0.02, and your alpha is 0.05. You therefore reject the null hypothesis and conclude that there is difference between the mean systolic blood pressures of these three racial groups. When you report these results, you need to include what the means are for each group and that there is a statistical difference.

You cannot conclude from this test alone where the statistically significant difference may lie. Perhaps group 2 was significantly greater than group 3 but not significantly greater than group 1. Perhaps there was a significant difference among all three groups. You would need to do further testing to draw that conclusion. This test merely lets you conclude that there is a difference among the average blood pressures of men from different racial groups.

If you really want to impress someone at your next Christmas party show them an analysis of variance test with only two groups (remember you could just do a *t*-test for that!) and then determine the *F*-ratio. If you take the square root, you have the *t*-value, which you could have determined by just doing a *t*-test on the two groups. It is statistically acceptable but not necessary to compute an *F*-ratio from an ANOVA test when there are only two groups and you will reach the same conclusion as you would using the t-test. All this might not be great dinner conversation, but it might come in handy the next time you are trying to discourage a boring hanger-on.

FROM THE STATISTICIAN   BRENDAN HEAVEY

Relationship Between Distributions

What is the relationship among chi-square analyses, *t*-tests, and *F*-tests? The following three facts might surprise you:

1. If an ANOVA analysis is performed on just two groups of subjects, the test gives the same results as a *t*-test.
2. The *t*-distribution, which is the underlying probability distribution of the *t*-test, looks almost identical to the normal distribution. In fact, the only difference is that it's a little flatter, with more probability assigned to the tails of the distribution.
3. An easy way to produce a chi-squared distribution is by summing the squares of a series of standard normal variables.

There are standard ways of converting among these distributions. The math is a bit higher level than we want to discuss here, but it's certainly doable. The process is called *transformation*. Some transformations are quite simple, like the square root transformation performed by taking the square root of every data point in a study variable. Other transformations are quite difficult and can involve formulas longer than a page.

Often, students feel discouraged in introductory statistics classes because they have a difficult time with the properties of distributions and the relationships between them. If you choose to go on to another statistics course (or if you are forced to take another one because of degree requirements), keep in mind the fact that they are all related. Perhaps this insight will give you a bit more motivation to understand their intricacies.

You can choose from an unlimited number of probability distributions. They all must have a total sum of probability, or area under the curve, equal to 1. Whenever you have to deal with a new one, just remember the five-step process for statistical testing, and you should be all right. In fact, you can do a surprising amount of decent statistical analyses by learning how to use a basic statistical software package like SPSS. You can thank the great statistical minds that came before us, like Pearson, RA Fisher, and Samuel Gosset for figuring out all the equations for you!

Appropriate Use of ANOVA

Several assumptions should be met before you use ANOVA.

- First, the samples must be independent (ideally random), and the measure must be at the interval or ratio level.
- The sample should have a normal distribution. But remember the central limit theorem. Because we are comparing means,

we can comfortably assume normality. The distribution of the original population doesn't matter; the means will be normally distributed.

- The last assumption is homogeneity of variance, which also isn't terribly concerning at this level because ANOVA still works pretty well even if this assumption isn't met.

So the big takeaway message about assumptions and ANOVA is that you need independent samples with an outcome or dependent variable at the interval or ratio level. You don't have to be concerned about the other assumptions too much. You should know about them because you will see your statistics computing program assess them (Norman & Streiner, 2008).

Repeat-Measures ANOVA

ANOVA has another really exciting application. (I can see you jumping out of your seats with excitement now!) But please remain calm. It is called **repeat-measures ANOVA**, and it is useful for dependent samples. You will see this application used frequently in nursing literature that examines a change over time in the same sample population. For example, suppose you want to compare the mean BMI of a group of children who participated in a 12-week after-school basketball program and a comparison group who did not. BMI becomes your dependent variable, and you are going to measure it, in each of the subjects and the controls, before the subjects begin the program, halfway through the program, and upon completion of the program. You can also design a study appropriate for repeat-measures ANOVA by taking the same group of subjects and measuring their weights before any intervention, then giving them three different weight control interventions, one at a time with two weeks per intervention. You then measure their weights before and after each intervention. By repeating the measures on the same group of subjects, you create a level of control over differences among the participants and make it easier to isolate the differences resulting from your intervention. You thus increase the likelihood that you will find statistically significant results when they exist. In effect, you increase the (can you hear the drum roll here?) **power** of the study (or the ability to detect a difference that really exists). You saw that coming right?

Issues of Concern with Repeat-Measures ANOVA

Repeat-measure ANOVA can be very helpful in decreasing not only the individual variation error, but also the required sample size needed to find a significant result. This is particularly helpful when it is difficult to recruit subjects or when funding is difficult to obtain.

However, all researchers using this method need to be aware of a couple of concerns:

- **Position or latency effects** occur when a subject is being exposed to more than one treatment over time and order of the treatment received impacts the outcome. For example, let's say you have a cancer study which includes treatment with surgery and chemotherapy. If surgically removing the cancerous tumor improves the ability of the chemotherapy to eliminate any remaining cancer cells, subjects who start with the surgery, followed by the chemotherapy, may experience a greater effect than those who start with the chemotherapy followed by the surgery. You can address this concern by randomly assigning the order of the interventions.
- **Carry-over effects** occur when previous treatments continue to have an effect through the next treatment. In this case, the measurement of the outcome or dependent variable after a particular treatment does not just reflect the impact of that treatment but rather includes the additional effect from the previous treatment as well. For example, if subjects in a weight study take a diet pill with a long half-life, they may need a "wash-out" period before beginning the next intervention to avoid having the effect of two interventions at the same time (Plichta & Garzon, 2009).

Appropriate Use of Repeat-Measures ANOVA

Like all other statistical techniques, appropriate use of repeat-measures ANOVA involves meeting some basic assumptions. The assumptions are the same as those for ANOVA, but there is one more—compound symmetry. **Compound symmetry** means that the measurements are correlated and of equal variances. So, if you are measuring BMI three times, the three results should be correlated with each other and approximately the same. **Homogeneity of variance** should also still be present and is the term used to indicate that those correlated BMI measurements need to have approximately equal variances.

The good news is that, once again, your statistical computing package will check all of this for you! If you look at your SPSS output, you will see an area for Mauchly's sphericity test. If this test is not significant you can tell the assumption of compound symmetry is met and can proceed with your analysis confidently (Munro, 2005). What on earth did we do before SPSS? Okay, I have to admit, I remember—and it wasn't pretty.

FROM THE STATISTICIAN   BRENDAN HEAVEY

Methods: Calculating an F-Statistic

An analysis of variance is a lot like a *t*-test extended to multiple groups of data. It's a little more difficult to understand conceptually, but in my opinion well worth the effort to learn! In fact, if you don't use ANOVA, you sometimes have to do a whole series of *t*-tests, and that can quickly increase the error associated with your analysis.

Let's say we have two variables; one is continuous and one is categorical. The categorical variable has three levels, and we're interested in looking at the mean value of the continuous variable in each of these categories. (See Figure 10-1.) Each of the three cells in the table has its own mean, which is identified using the Greek letter μ (mu). (Don't ask me why we use ancient Greek; we follow the mathematicians lead on this.) Attached to each μ character is a subscript that indicates the number of the group from which the mean is determined. The overall mean (or grand mean) is denoted by a period (μ.). In ANOVA, we're always interested in a null hypothesis that makes all of the individual cell means equal to each other.

Figure 10-1 Beginning of General ANOVA Table.

	Level 1	Level 2	Level 3	Grand Mean
Variable	μ_1	μ_2	μ_3	μ.

To perform a test of this hypothesis, we compute an *F*-statistic (named after R.A. Fisher, who developed ANOVA). The *F*-statistic is simply a ratio of variances. (Remember, variance is just a measure of how a set of values differs from a single value.) The first variance component in an *F*-statistic is derived from the variance of the cell means around the grand mean (this is the variance between the groups). The second variance component in an *F*-statistic is derived from how each individual data point differs from its respective cell mean (this is the variance within the group itself).

FROM THE STATISTICIAN   BRENDAN HEAVEY

Let's look at an example. We will revisit the data we looked at from the *t*-test FTS (Chapter 9). The data was collected on trauma cases aged 25 and under during one 72-hour period at an upstate New York tertiary care facility. In that FTS, we compared the mean age between groups who had a positive drug screen and those who did not. Now we are interested to see whether the mean age of a patient differs among the classes of injury the patients had treated. The data is presented in Figure 10-2.

Figure 10-2 Age and Injury Level for Patients Seen in a 72-Hour Period at a Trauma Center.

Age	Injury	Age	Injury
2	2	20	1
3	2	20	2
5	0	20	2
7	1	20	2
8	2	22	2
15	2	22	2
15	2	23	1
18	2	23	1
19	1	25	0
19	2	25	2

The first step is to get our data to look like the generalized table (Figure 10-3):

Figure 10-3 Beginning of General ANOVA Table.

	Factor Level 1	Factor Level 2	Factor Level 3	Grand Mean
Variable	μ_1	μ_2	μ_3	$\mu.$

Here's how our data looks in the general ANOVA table (Figure 10-4):

Figure 10-4 Our Data in the General ANOVA Table.

	No Injury	Minor Injury	Major Injury
Age	5, 25	7, 19, 20, 23, 23	2 ,2, 8, 15, 15, 18, 19, 20, 20, 21, 22, 22, 25

(continues)

FROM THE STATISTICIAN · BRENDAN HEAVEY

Now we solve for the unknown parameters:

$$\mu_1 = \frac{5+25}{2} = 15$$

$$\mu_2 = \frac{7+19+20+23+23}{5} = 18.4$$

$$\mu_3 = \frac{2+2+8+15+15+18+19+20+20+21+22+22+25}{13} = 16.08$$

$$\mu. = \frac{5+25+7+19+20+23+23+2+2+8+15+15+18+19+20+20+21+22+22+25}{20} = 16.6$$

In this hypothesis, our null hypothesis is:

H_0: The three cell means, $\mu_1 = 15$, $\mu_2 = 18.4$, $\mu_3 = 16.08$, are equal.

The alternative hypothesis is:

H_1: They are not *all* equal.

The results of the ANOVA are shown in Figure 10-5. The *p*-value for this test is 0.823, derived from the *F*-statistic value of 0.198. Assuming an alpha of 0.05, this *p*-value indicates that there is not enough evidence to reject the null hypothesis.

Figure 10-5 Statistical Program Output: ANOVA Table.

ANOVA

Age

	Sum of Squares	*df*	Mean Square	F	Significance
Between groups	23.908	2	11.954	0.198	0.823
Within groups	1028.892	17	60.523		
Total	1052.800	19			

Where does the *F*-statistic value come from? It is the mean square between groups divided by the mean square within groups or, using data from Figure 10-5:

$$F = \frac{11.954}{60.523} = 0.198$$

Where do the mean squares come from? These are just the sums of squares divided by their respective degrees of freedom.

FROM THE STATISTICIAN   BRENDAN HEAVEY

Look at Figure 10-5, and you can see that the following is true:

$$\frac{23.908}{2} = 11.954 \qquad \frac{1028.892}{17} = 60.523$$

Now we reach the big question: Where do the sums of squares come from? They are the measurements of the variance components from two different sources:

- How much the cell means vary around the grand mean.
- How much the individual data points vary around their respective cell means.

The analysis of variance compares these two measures to derive the F-statistic.

If you want to see ANOVA in action, check out the articles by Chen et al. (2007), Papastavrou et al. (2009), and Zurmehly (2008).

Summary

You are doing a spectacular job at learning these concepts if you made it this far! Let's review the main points from this chapter.

The ANOVA (analysis of variance) is used when comparing the sample means for a single dependent variable among two or more independent groups or samples.

The repeat-measures ANOVA is used to examine a change over time in the same sample population. The test is useful for dependent samples. When using repeat-measures ANOVA, you must be aware of position or latency effects.

These effects can occur when a subject is being exposed to more then one treatment over time and the order of the treatments received can impact the outcome in different ways. Also, be aware of carry-over effects, which occur when previous treatments continue to have an effect through the next treatment and the measurement of the dependent variable may not be accurate.

Take a moment to rest your brain before moving on to the next chapter! You have only two more chapters to go. Isn't the information in the beginning chapters starting to look easy now? This will too; it just takes time.

CHAPTER 10 REVIEW QUESTIONS

Questions 1–12: In a study by Vassiliadou et al. (2008), the role of nursing in sexual counseling of myocardial patients was examined. The authors examined professional nurses and collected data about their gender, age, education, unit of employment, and experience in cardiac clinics. They then compared, among other things, the knowledge and comfort level nurses had with regard to sexual counseling. [Reprinted with permission from *The Health Sciences Journal*. Original source is Vassiliadou et al. (2008).]

1. What are the dependent variables?

   _____

   _____

2. If knowledge is measured by the score in points the nurse receives on a test, is this a quantitative or qualitative variable? Continuous or categorical? What level of measurement is it?

   _____

   _____

   _____

3. These researchers conducted surveys at a nursing conference. What type of sample is this? How does this affect generalizability of the results?

   _____

   _____

4. Write an appropriate null hypothesis.

   _____

5. Write an appropriate alternative hypothesis.

   _____

6. The study has an alpha of 0.05 and a power of 80%. They found a relationship between the unit the nurses worked on and the knowledge scores with a *p*-value of 0.01. What should they conclude?

   _____

7. When comparing nurses from different units and their comfort with this type of counseling, they found a *p*-value of > 0.17. What should they conclude about the comfort level of nurses from different units?

   _____

8. When comparing nurses from different units and their comfort level with this type of counseling ($p > 0.17$), what is the F-value probably close to?

9. If this conclusion is incorrect, what type of error would the researchers be making?

10. What is the probability of making this type of error?

11. If the researchers think this type of error is occurring, what might they do to fix it?

12. Why is ANOVA an appropriate test for this study?

Questions 13–21: A study by Heyman et al. (2008) examined a sample of 245 elderly individuals living in long-term care facilities. Each had a grade II–IV pressure ulcer. The pressure ulcers were examined at enrollment and then again at 3 and 9 weeks. All of the patients received standard care plus an additional nutritional supplement. The goal of the study was to examine the effects of the nutritional supplement plus routine care on the healing of pressure ulcers in long-term care patients. (See Figure 10-6.)

13. What is the dependent variable?

14. What is the independent variable?

15. What level of measurement is the dependent variable?

16. Is it qualitative or quantitative?

17. Is it continuous or categorical?

18. Is the sample independent or dependent?

(continues)

19. All subjects who met eligibility requirements and consented at 61 long-term care facilities were enrolled with no exclusion criteria. What type of sampling method is this?

20. Write an appropriate null hypothesis.

21. Write an appropriate alternative hypothesis.

Questions 22–31: Look at Figure 10-6.

22. This study has an alpha of 0.05 and a power of 0.80. Was the size of the pressure ulcer at the first follow-up (visit 2) significantly different from the size at visit 1?

23. Was the size of the pressure ulcer significantly different at the 9-week follow up (visit 3)?

24. What would you conclude regarding your null hypothesis?

25. If type of error could you be making?

26. What is your chance of making this type of error?

27. As the nurse manager in a long-term care facility, you believe these results are clinically significant. What recommendation would you make in terms of clinical care?

28. Why is repeat-measures ANOVA an appropriate choice for analysis?

29. By using this sample as their own control group, these researchers were able to minimize the effect of differences among the participants and see the effect of the intervention more clearly. This increased what in the study?

   _____

30. Using the participants as their own controls minimized the effect of the differences among the participants. How does this affect the sample size needed?

   _____

31. Any researcher using repeat-measures ANOVA needs to be aware of position and carry-over effects. What are these? Are they a concern in this study?

   _____

   _____

   _____

Figure 10-6 Reduction in Mean Pressure Ulcer Area Achieved with the Oral Nutritional Supplement.

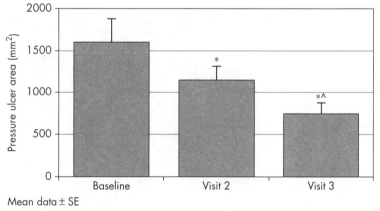

Mean data ± SE
* $p < 0.0001$ compared with baseline; ^$p < 0.0001$ compared with week 3, visit 2

CHAPTER 10 FTS REVIEW QUESTION

32. You are asked to evaluate a nursing program's admission criteria and want to determine whether the mean GPA is different for individuals with higher-ranked letters of recommendation (on a 5-point scale, 1 = poor, 5 = excellent). You develop the following ANOVA table:

ANOVA

GPA

	Sum of Squares	*df*	Mean Square	F	Significance
Between groups	0.686	4			0.316
Within groups	12.122	85			
Total	12.807	89			

Complete the calculations necessary to fill in the rest of the table. What do you conclude?

Use your computer to practice these applications.

The companion website for this book has a computer-based application example for this material. Check it out!

Analyze	Graphs	Utilities	Add-ons	Window	Help

Reports ▶

Descriptive Statistics ▶

Tables ▶

Compare Means ▶ | M Means...

General Linear Model ▶ | One-Sample T Test...

Generalized Linear Models ▶ | Independent-Samples T Test...

Mixed Models ▶ | Paired-Samples T Test...

Correlate ▶

Regression ▶ | One-Way ANOVA...

ANSWERS TO CHAPTER 10 REVIEW QUESTIONS

1. Knowledge and comfort level

3. Nonprobability convenience sample; may not be representative; may be a more educated group of nurses or a particularly interested group of nurses

5. Answers may vary. For example, H_1: There is a difference in the knowledge level of nurses working on different units.

7. Fail to reject the null, there is no significant difference.

9. Type two

11. Increase the sample size

13. Pressure ulcer size

15. Collected as ratio level data, analyzed as ordinal level data

17. Continuous

19. Nonprobability, convenience sampling

21. Answers may vary. For example, H_1: Pressure ulcers decrease in size by 9 weeks.

23. Yes

25. Type one

27. To give the nutritional supplement

29. Power

31. Position effects (if the order of the interventions affects the outcome) can be avoided by random assignment), and carry-over effects need a wash-out period. Since this study had only one intervention, these are not a concern.

Chapter 11

Correlation Coefficients

What about looking for a relationship between two variables in the same sample?

OBJECTIVES

By the end of this chapter students will be able to:

- Identify situations in which using a correlation coefficient is appropriate.

- Compare correlation coefficients and determine when the requirements of each are met.

- Appropriately match the level of measurement of a variable and the appropriate correlation coefficient test.

- Write null and alternative hypotheses that demonstrate an understanding of the guiding principles of correlation coefficients.

- Evaluate a correlation coefficient, and assess the direction of the relationship.

- Differentiate between the strength and the direction of the relationship.

- Determine whether a correlation is statistically significant.

- Identify and calculate the percentage of variance.

- Explain in plain English what the percentage of variance means, and prepare a public health headline using this information.

- Read and interpret a computer printout with correlation coefficients, identifying whether the correlation coefficient is statistically significant, the direction of the relationship and the strength of the relationship, and stating these results in statistical terms and in plain English.

- Critique a current nursing research article that uses correlation coefficients, interpret the results statistically and in plain English, and prepare a public health report using this information.

KEY TERMS

Chi-square test
The test used to find a relationship or difference in an outcome or dependent variable
measured at the nominal or ordinal level.

Coefficient of determination
The square of Pearson's *r* (r^2).

Correlation
A relationship between at least two variables.

Direction of the relationship
Either the positive or the negative nature of
the relationship. If positive, both variables
move in the same direction; if negative,
when one variable increases in value the
other decreases, and vice versa.

Homoscedasticity
Equal spread of one variable around all the
levels of another variable.

Pearson's correlation coefficient (r)
The test used if you are looking for a relationship
between two variables that are normally distributed and at the interval or ratio level.

Percentage of variance
The amount of variance in one variable that is
explained by the second variable, determined
by multiplying the coefficient of determination
by 100

Spearman correlation coefficient (ρ)
The test used if you are looking for a relationship
between two variables and at least one is ordinal or not normally distributed.

Strength of the relationship
Determined by the absolute value of the correlation coefficient.

Looking for a Relationship in One Sample

Chapters 8–10 focused on how to determine
whether there are statistically significant differences in an outcome variable from two or more
samples. These tests, however, don't always
answer the researcher's question. Sometimes
nurses want to know the relationship or association between two variables in a single sample.
For example, is there an association between
working overtime hours and medication errors
among the nurses in your hospital?

The Null and Alternative Hypotheses

In this example, you would develop the following null and alternative hypotheses.

H_0: There is no association between overtime hours worked and medication errors.

H_1: There is an association between overtime hours worked and medication errors.

When they did this very study in New York,
they found a statistically significant positive

relationship between overtime hours worked and medication errors; so they rejected the null hypothesis. The public health laws were changed as a result, and it is now illegal in New York State to mandate a nurse to work overtime beyond a 16-hour shift. Nurses who work shifts longer than this voluntarily (or for the extra income) are held personally responsible for any errors they make due to fatigue or exhaustion (New York State Nurses Association, n.d.). This is an example of looking for a relationship, or **correlation**, between two variables, in this case, hours worked and medication errors.

Selecting the Best Correlation Test to Use

For the several types of correlation tests, the lead question is the same as it was before: What level of measurement are my variables? (Now you understand why that question was in the first chapter!) If in the relationship you wish to examine, at least one of the variables is only measured at a nominal level, you still need to use the **chi-square test**, but this time you are looking at a relationship between two variables from only one independent sample. (What a flexible test!) However:

- If the lowest level of data collected for at least one variable is measured at the ordinal level or is not normally distributed, you should use the **Spearman correlation coefficient** (ρ, rho). (You can sometimes use the Pearson's correlation coefficient with ordinal data too, but that is a long story, and you don't need to worry about now.)
- If you have two variables that are at the interval or ratio data level and are normally distributed, you can use the **Pearson's correlation coefficient** (r).

Direction of the Relationship

Both the Spearman and Pearson's correlation coefficients describe the direction and strength of a linear relationship between two variables. A linear association is represented by a straight line. The **direction of the relationship** is either positive or negative. A positive correlation means that, when one variable increases, the other variable does too and that when one decreases, so does the other. Both variables move in the same direction. In a positive correlation, the coefficient (ρ or r) is positive. Let's use every professor's favorite example of a positive relationship. (Yes, we do this for subliminal messaging effect as well.) The relationship between the time spent studying for an exam and the grade received on the exam is usually positively correlated. Conversely, if less time is spent on studying, the grade received is usually lower.

In a negative relationship or correlation, if one variable increases, the second variable decreases and vice versa. For example, the relationship between smoking and life expectancy has a negative correlation. When smoking increases, life expectancy decreases; when smoking decreases, life expectancy increases. In this case, the correlation coefficient (ρ or r) is negative.

Sample Size

You must have a sample of at least three subjects for correlation coefficients. If you are looking for a linear relationship between only two measures (subjects) of a variable, you will always find one: You can always connect two points with a straight line (that's why it's called linear). For all of these tests, you need two variables to correlate and at least three subjects in the sample; then you can compute the appropriate correlation coefficient.

Strength of the Relationship

The **strength of the relationship** or correlation is determined by the absolute value of the correlation coefficient. Absolute value is just the numeric value of a number without the positive or negative indicator. For example, the absolute value of -4 is 4, and the absolute value of $+4$ is 4.

Correlation coefficients are always between -1 and $+1$.

- A correlation coefficient of -1 indicates a perfect negative relationship.
- The closer the correlation is to zero, the weaker the relationship is.
- If the correlation is zero, there is no relationship at all. In this case, the variables are completely independent.
- At the other extreme, a correlation coefficient of 1 indicates a perfect positive relationship.
- If the *absolute* value of the correlation coefficient is < 0.3, the relationship between the variables is weak.
- If it is 0.3–0.5, the relationship between the variables is moderate.
- If it is > 0.5, the relationship between the variables is strong.

So, for example, putting the direction and strength concepts together, a correlation coefficient of 0.2 shows a weak positive relationship between the variables. A correlation coefficient of -0.6 shows a strong negative relationship between the variables.

Statistical Significance

But wait a minute here, don't be fooled. You need to look at something else to determine whether these results are significant. What do you always need to check before you know whether the results are statistically significant?

YES—the *p*-value! Your statistical computing package will give you a corresponding *p*-value, which determines whether your correlation coefficient is significant. If your sample size is very small, you may have large correlation coefficients that are not significant ($p >$ alpha). Even small correlation coefficients can be significant when the sample is large ($p <$ alpha).

Nurses usually remember this quite well. I usually remind my class that the last step at the end of a nursing shift (tabulating the patient's intake and output for the shift) and the last step at the end of a statistics test are remarkably similar. You always have to check the "pee" value! You have to know the *p*-value before you are done with your statistical analysis as well.

Appropriate Use of Correlation Coefficients

Selecting any test depends on certain assumptions which for correlation coefficients should include the following:.

- First, the sample subjects should be independent and randomly selected.
- Second, the appropriate level of measurement should be met (if at least one variable is nominal, chi-square; if the lowest level of data is ordinal, Spearman's; if both variables are interval/ratio, Pearson's).
- Third, two variables must be compared, and a linear relationship must be present (you can always check a scatter plot to make sure this is the case).
- If you wish to use the Pearson's correlation coefficient, both variables should be normally distributed in the population (the fancy term for this is *bivariate normal*) and **homoscedasticity** should be present. Homoscedasticity can be seen visually on a scatter plot. It is a truly horrific word to try to say but its

meaning is pretty simple. If the spread of a variable is about the same around all the levels of another variable this assumption is met. For example, if as each hour of work increases there are 1-2 more nursing errors, homoscedasticity is present. However, if at 5 hours of work 0-3 errors are present, and at 10 hours of work 0–9 errors are reported, and at 15 hours of work 1–15 errors are reported, this assumption is violated. These last two assumptions for the Pearson's correlation coefficient can be violated if the sample size is large enough. The big takeaway message about these assumptions is to make sure your sample has at least 50 subjects. Then you can proceed as long as you have ratio/interval level data (Corty, 2007).

Here are some questions to answer before you select the best correlation test:

- Do you have one independent sample?
- Are you looking for a linear relationship between two variables in this sample?
- What is the lowest level of measurement for each of your variables?

    Nominal—select chi-square.

    Ordinal—select Spearman's.

    Interval/ratio—select Pearson's.

When selecting the correlation test, make sure your data meets the test's assumptions. If it does not, you need to select a test at a lower level. For example, if you wish to use Pearson's correlation coefficient but your sample is only 20 subjects and is not normally distributed, you generally need to use the Spearman's correlation coefficient.

More Uses for Pearson's *r*

You should know one other thing about the Pearson's *r*. If you square it (r^2), it becomes the **coefficient of determination**. If you then multiply it by 100, it tells you something called the **percentage of variance**, which nurses readily understand. The **percentage of variance** is simply the amount of variance in one variable that is explained by the second variable. For example, suppose you were reading a study that found that daily caloric intake and total serum cholesterol had a statistically significant Pearson's correlation coefficient of 0.7 ($r = 0.7$). You could square this number ($0.7 \times 0.7 = 0.49$) to calculate the coefficient of determination. When you multiply that coefficient by 100, you can then use English again: "Forty-nine percent of the differences they found in total serum cholesterol were explained by differences in daily caloric intake."

The other neat piece of information that you can determine with this percentage is the amount of the differences in total serum cholesterol that were related to factors other than daily caloric intake (e.g., genetics, exercise, etc.). That amount is the difference between the percentage of variance and 100%, in this case, $100\% - 49\% = 51\%$. In terms of clinical importance, any value of $r > 0.3$ (which you know means it explains about 9% of the variance) is considered clinically important (Grove, 2007). Now that is pretty understandable!

You can also use the Pearson's correlation coefficient (*r*) to determine the effect size to use when calculating sample size. Think about it; it makes sense. The effect size is just an estimate of the relationship/difference you are attempting to find.

- When you have a strong correlation, you have a large effect size and don't need such a large a sample to find a statistically significant difference if it exists.
- When the strength of the correlation is weak, the effect size is small and you need a larger sample to detect statistically significant differences.

For example, when Pearson's $r = 0.4$, one of your variables explains 16% of the variance in the other, which is considered a medium effect size. When Pearson's $r = 0.6$, one of your variables explains 36% of the variance of the other, which is a large effect size. You will need a larger sample to detect the small or medium correlation (i.e., $r = 0.4$) and a smaller sample when you are trying to detect the large correlation (i.e., $r = 0.6$). (I told you it made sense.)

FROM THE STATISTICIAN   BRENDAN HEAVEY

Methods: Correlation Coefficients

Here's an example of how to use correlation coefficients. The director of the local community center believes that students are at increased risk for accidental injury as they progress through the higher grades in high school. He wants to know how these two variables (increased risk of accidental injury and grade level) are related in the population that the center serves. He gives you a database with randomly collected surveys of 108 adolescents who participate at the center and asks you to complete an analysis. You note two questions in particular: One asks the student to identify his or her current grade, and another asks how often the student experienced an accidental injury in the last six months. Injury risk is ranked on a 1–5 scale: 1 = never, 2 = less than three times, 3 = three to five times, 4 = five to seven times, 5 = more than seven times. You decide to analyze these two variables using a correlation coefficient. Being the statistical genius that you are, you know that identifying the correct correlation coefficient for the job means answering a few questions.

First, do you have one independent sample? In this example, the data you have is all collected from adolescents at one community center. There is no contrasting sample, and you are not dividing the sample into different samples to compare. Each of the adolescents was surveyed only once, and they are not related in any way. Therefore, you have one independent sample.

Second, you need to be sure that you are looking for a linear relationship between two variables and you are.

Last, you must identify the level of measurement of the variables in order to select the correct correlation coefficient. The first variable is the current grade level of the student, which is interval/ratio level. The level of measurement of the risk scale is ordinal.

You can now identify which correlation coefficient is appropriate for this sample. Your statistical program outputs these tables in Figures 11-1 and 11-2. Which table is appropriate for your analysis and why?

Because you know your risk scale variable is ordinal, you know you must use the Spearman ρ correlation coefficient in Figure 11-2. (If it were interval or ratio, you could use the table in Figure 11-1 and the Pearson's correlation coefficient.) Looking at Figure 11-2, you can determine that the correlation between the risk of injury and the student's grade level is actually 0.156. You, of course, also know that the p-value associated with this correlation is 0.106, which is not significant. You are then able to report to the community center director that, unfortunately, the grade level explains only 2.4% (0.156 × 0.156) of the variance in accidental injury in this sample. It is not significantly related to the risk for accidental injury.

FROM THE STATISTICIAN   BRENDAN HEAVEY

Before you wrap this analysis up, go back to Figure 11-2 and make sure you understand what the other numbers mean. Don't worry—they're pretty straightforward. First, you know that $N = 108$ means that 108 adolescents were in your sample. But why is 1.00 listed as the correlation coefficient between grade and grade and between risk and risk? That number shows that, when you correlate a variable with itself, the correlation coefficient is 1.00. It's a perfect correlation. Any variable should correlate perfectly with itself!

Figure 11-1 Correlation Coefficient: Table 1.

Correlations

		Risk	Grade
Risk	Pearson's correlation	1.000	0.159
	Significance (2-tailed)		0.101
	N	108.000	108
Grade	Pearson Correlation	0.159	1.000
	Significance (2-tailed)	0.101	
	N	108	108.000

Figure 11-2 Correlation Coefficient: Table 2.

			Risk	Grade
Spearman's ρ	Risk	Correlation Coefficient	1.000	0.156
		Significance (2-tailed)	.	0.106
		N	108	108
	Grade	Correlation Coefficient	0.156	1.000
		Significance (2-tailed)	0.106	.
		N	108	108

Summary

Good job completing Chapter 11! Now we will review the concepts.

A correlation is the relationship between two variables.

- We use the chi-square test to look for a correlation when you have an independent sample and at least one of the variables you wish to examine is of nominal-level data.
- The Spearman correlation coefficient is used if the variable with the lowest level of data is ordinal or not normally distributed.
- If you have two normally distributed interval or ratio level variables, the Pearson's correlation coefficient is used.

Both the Spearman and Pearson's correlation coefficients tell you the direction and strength of the linear relationship between the two variables. The direction of the relationship can be either positive or negative. In a positive correlation, as one variable increases, so does the other; as one variable decreases, so does the other. In a negative correlation, as one variable increases, the second variable decreases; as one variable decreases, the second increases.

The strength of the relationship is determined by the absolute value of the correlation coefficient. The coefficient of determination is represented by r^2 because you must square Pearson's r. The percentage of variance is the amount of variance in one variable that is explained by the second variable, and it is determined by multiplying the coefficient of determination (r^2) by 100.

These concepts may be a little confusing. So review this chapter until you feel completely confident. Keep your head up and continue to study hard. Believe it or not, the concepts eventually sink in as you continue to use them. Do you remember learning how to take a blood pressure? I thought I'd never master the skill, and I felt very, very anxious. Now blood pressures are old hat. Statistics is the same; you just need to practice until the concepts make sense. The more you use them, the clearer they become.

CHAPTER 11 REVIEW QUESTIONS

Questions 1–18: You are asked to conduct a study to determine whether there is an association between consumption of milk proteins and levels of serum antibodies in children with autism. You randomly select 50 children previously enrolled in an autism clinical trial, and they are the sample for the study. You select an alpha of 0.05 and a power of 0.80.

1. Your study measures consumption of milk proteins as a yes-or-no question. It measures serum antibodies as a present-or-not-present question. What level are the two variables?

_____

2. What analysis method do you propose based on this information?

_____

3. Your research partner believes it would be better to measure milk protein consumption as a low/moderate/high question and to quantify the serum antibody level by using the actual amount present. If you take this approach, what– analysis method do you propose?

_____

4. The biostatistician in your department recommends you change your milk protein measurement to one that is the number of servings per day. You continue to use the actual quantity of the serum antibodies. You might now recommend what analysis method?

_____

5. Write an appropriate null hypothesis for this study.

_____

6. Write an appropriate alternative hypothesis for this study.

_____

7. Is your sample size large enough to conduct a correlation test? Is it large enough to assume a normal distribution and homoscedasticity?

_____

8. You decide to utilize the measurement variables as recommended by the biostatistician and conduct a Pearson's correlation coefficient test. You determine $r = 0.6$. What must your p-value be for this to be statistically significant?

_____

9. Your p-value is 0.08. Is this significant?

_____

10. What do you conclude?

_____

11. Suppose that you were able to refine your measurement tools and repeat the study and that you determine you had an $r = 0.6$ with a p-value of 0.049, what would you conclude?

_____

12. This information would let you know that your original conclusion was actually what type of error?

(continues)

13. What is the strength of the relationship between consumption of milk proteins and serum antibodies?

_____

14. Is the relationship positive or negative? Interpret this in English.

_____

15. In this study, what percentage of variance in serum antibody levels is explained by the consumption of milk proteins in children with autism?

_____

16. How much of the variance is explained by other variables?

_____

17. Is this clinically important?

_____

18. If you were going to use this effect size to determine your sample size for another study, would you expect to need a large or small sample?

_____

Questions 19–24: You develop a screening test to be used for children with autism to detect serum antibodies from milk protein consumption and have the following 2 × 2 table.

	+ disease	No disease	Totals
Positive test	10	2	12
Negative test	3	220	223
Totals	13	222	235

Calculate the following values:

19. Sensitivity:

_____

20. Specificity:

_____

21. Positive predictive value:

22. Negative predictive value:

23. Prevalence:

24. If early treatment helps, is this a good screen?

*Questions 25–27:*You are asked to complete a study for a small school district that is trying to keep as many students at age-appropriate grade levels as possible. You have a measure of grade level and age for the students, as well as the following statistical programming output from a randomized independent sample.

Correlations

		Age	Grade
Age	Pearson correlation	1.000	0.382*
	Significance (2-tailed)		0.000
	N	108.000	108
Grade	Pearson correlation	0.382*	1.000
	Significance (2-tailed)	0.000	
	N	108	108.000

*Correlation is significant at the 0.01 level (2-tailed).

Correlations

			Age	Grade
Spearman's ρ	Age	Correlation coefficient	1.000	0.378*
		Significance (2-tailed)	.	0.000
		N	108	108
	Grade	Correlation coefficient	0.378*	1.000
		Significance (2-tailed)	0.000	.
		N	108	108

*Correlation is significant at the 0.01 level (2-tailed).

(continues)

25. What is your sample size?

_____

26. What is the appropriate correlation coefficient and why?

_____

27. Are age and grade significantly correlated?

_____

Use your computer to practice these applications.

The companion website for this book has a computer-based application example for this material. Check it out!

Analyze	Graphs	Utilities	Add-ons	Window
Reports	▶			
Descriptive Statistics	▶			
Tables	▶			
Compare Means	▶		ht	
General Linear Model	▶			
Generalized Linear Models	▶			
Mixed Models	▶		66.12182052	
Correlate	▶		Bivariate...	

ANSWERS TO CHAPTER 11 REVIEW QUESTIONS

1. Both nominal

3. Ordinal/ratio—Spearman's correlation coefficient

5. H_0: There is no association between milk protein consumption and serum antibodies.

7. Yes, it is greater than or equal to 3; yes, it is greater than or equal to 50.

9. No

11. Reject the null; there is a relationship.

13. 0.6 = strong

15. $0.6 \times 0.6 = 0.36 = 36\%$

17. Yes, $> 9\%$

19. $10 \div 13$

21. $10 \div 12$

23. $13 \div 235$

25. 108 students

27. $r = 0.382$, which is significant ($p < 0.01$)

Relative Risk, Odds Ratio, and Attributable Risk

Making the public announcement.

OBJECTIVES

By the end of this chapter students will be able to:

- Define epidemiology.

- Compare and contrast the three major study designs used in epidemiology, and evaluate the strengths and weaknesses of each.

- Compare and contrast incidence data and prevalence data.

- Explain why relative risk is a helpful measure.

- Write null and alternative hypotheses that demonstrate an understanding of relative risk (RR) and the odds ratio (OR).

- Formulate a 2×2 table from a given data set.

- Calculate incident rates, relative risk, and odds ratios.

- Interpret relative risks and odds ratios of less than one, equal to one, and greater than one.

- Evaluate whether it is appropriate to calculate a relative risk or an odds ratio from three nursing research proposals.

- Calculate the attributable risk for the exposed group, and interpret it for the exposed group in statistical terms and in plain English.

- Prepare a public health headline that states attributable risk results in language the general population will understand.

(continues)

- Critique a current nursing research article that utilizes odds ratios, and interpret the results statistically and in plain English.
- Prepare a public health report using odds ratio results in language the general public will understand.
- Interpret SPSS output, and determine whether a given relative risk and odds ratio are significant. Explain these results statistically and in plain English.

KEY TERMS

Attributable risk for the exposed group (AR_e)
The amount of a disease or outcome in an exposed group that is due to a particular exposure.

Case control study
A study design that starts with the outcome of interest and looks back to determine exposure.

Cohort study
A prospective design that follows a group of individuals over time to see who develops the outcome of interest.

Cross-sectional study
A study design that collects the data about exposure and outcome at the same time.

Epidemiology
The study of the distribution of disease.

Incidence cases
The number of new cases that occur among your sample during the duration of the study.

Odds ratio (OR)
Calculates an approximation of the relative risk using prevalence data (odds that a case was exposed divided by the odds that a control was exposed).

Prevalence cases
Those cases that already exist in a population.

Protective effect
When an exposure helps prevent a disease (a significant relative risk of less than one).

Relative risk (RR)
The incidence rate in the exposed sample divided by the incidence rate of those not exposed.

Relative risk of one
There is no association between the exposure and the illness.

Risk factor
An exposure that is associated with increased rates of disease.

Risk ratio
Another name for relative risk.

Epidemiology

Nursing is overlapping more and more with **epidemiology**, which is actually the study of the distribution of disease (Gordis, 2000). (Many people, including a number in the medical profession who should know better, have no idea what epidemiology is. Although I have a doctorate in epidemiology, on multiple occasions I have been introduced as an endocrinologist!) Epidemiologists like to see how disease is distributed and then ask the age-old question: Why? Some of the tools we use to examine these questions in the public health arena are becoming more and more popular in nursing research. So I am going to devote a whole chapter to making sure you are ready to combine what you know as a nurse with what you can learn in this chapter.

Study Designs Used in Epidemiology

There are basically three types of epidemiological studies (and many hybrid versions of them that you don't have to worry about right now):

- Cohort study
- Case control
- Cross-sectional

Cohort Study

A **cohort study** is a prospective design that follows a group of individuals over time to see who develops the outcome of interest.

For example, you might follow the nurses at your hospital to see which, if any, develops osteoporosis. In a cohort study, you start by measuring exposure, and then you monitor for outcomes. In this study, the exposure you are measuring is consumption of dairy products, and you are monitoring for the outcome of osteoporosis.

You also have to eliminate the **prevalence cases**, that is, the nurses who already have the disease you wish to study. Then you conduct an initial survey of the remaining nurses to see what they eat and drink, whether they smoke, whether they lift patients regularly, what unit they work on, how many hours they sleep, and so on. You then monitor the group for 40 years and see who develops osteoporosis, your outcome of interest. You can also look at multiple exposures (diet, smoking, lifting, sleeping, etc.) and determine which, if any, are associated with developing osteoporosis later in life.

One of the advantages of this type of study is that you can monitor for **incidence cases**, which are the new cases that occur among your sample during the duration of your study. That enables you to calculate something called a **relative risk (RR)**, the incidence rate in the exposed sample divided by the incidence rate of those not exposed. The relative risk is also sometimes referred to as the **risk ratio**.

Suppose, for example, in your sample of, say, 300 nurses, you found that, of the 100 nurses who consumed three servings of dairy products daily, only 4 developed osteoporosis. At the same time, among the 200 nurses who did not consume three servings of dairy products daily, 20 developed osteoporosis. We can make a 2×2 table to help sort out the results (see Figure 12-1).

The incidence cases are all the nurses who developed osteoporosis during the 40-year span of your study: $A + C = 24$. The incidence rate is simply the incidence cases divided by the whole sample times 100: in this case, $24 \div 300 \times 100 = 8\%$. This calculation tells you that 8% of your sample developed osteoporosis during the course of your study. You now need to

Figure 12-1 Consumption of Three Dairy Products (Exposure) and Osteoporosis Disease (Disease).

	Disease	**No disease**	**Total**
Exposed	$A = 4$	$B = 96$	$A + B = 100$
Not exposed*	$C = 20$	$D = 180$	$C + D = 200$
Total	$A + C = 24$	$B + D = 276$	$A + B + C + D = 300$

*Did not consume three dairy products a day.

compare the incidence in the exposed sample to the incidence in the nonexposed sample. This is the relative risk (RR). The formula is:

$$RR = \frac{\frac{A}{A + B}}{\frac{C}{C + D}}$$

where

A = subjects with the exposure and the disease
B = subjects with the exposure and without the disease
C = subjects without the exposure but with the disease
D = subjects without the exposure and without the disease

The calculation in this case is:

$$RR = \frac{\frac{4}{100}}{\frac{20}{200}} = \frac{0.4}{0.1}, \text{ or } 40\%$$

The interpretation of this result is that those who were exposed (consumed three servings of dairy a day) were less than half as likely (40% as likely) to develop osteoporosis later in life as those who were not exposed (didn't consume three servings of dairy). In this case, the exposure may have had a **protective effect** on dis-

ease development. A significant relative risk of less than one indicates a protective effect is associated with the exposure.

Other interpretations are possible:

• A **relative risk of one** indicates that there is no association between the exposure and the illness. For example, you may have found that consuming two cups of fruit juice had no effect on future osteoporosis development; this finding would be reflected by a relative risk of approximately one. The incidence of the disease is the same in the group that was exposed and in the group that was not.

• If the relative risk is greater than one, the group that was exposed has a higher incidence rate than the group that was not. So the exposure may be a **risk factor** for the development of the disease. For example, suppose in your study you found that the relative risk for smokers was 5.0. This number means that the incidence rate for osteoporosis was five times higher for smokers than for nonsmokers. Put a little differently, those who smoked were five times as likely to develop osteoporosis.

Don't ever forget that, even with a relative risk as high as 5.0, you still need to see whether the number is statistically significant. Statistical significance of the relative risk is once again determined by the *p*-value of the associated chi-square test. You always need to check the *p*.

Case Control Study

A cohort study sounds great, but what about when you can't get a grant to cover the cost of a 40-year prospective trial? Or you are trying to finish a dissertation in less than 40 years? Or do you want to examine a disease that is incredibly rare and may not even show up in a sample of 300 even if you follow them for 40 years? Another study design frequently used in epidemiology, especially when funding is tight or the disease is rare, is called a **case control study**. This type of study starts with the outcome of interest (the disease) and looks back to determine exposure. For example, 10 patients in your hospital have a rapidly progressing case of respiratory failure. All 10 were relatively healthy adults until developing symptoms that included fever and a cough.

You may start your study with this as your sample population (seven cases with similar unusual symptoms) and look back to determine what they may have been exposed to. You interview the patients and their families, review their medical records, and collect data on food consumed, recent travel, occupational exposures, previous illnesses, sexual partners, drug use, living situations. You also obtain biological specimens. Unfortunately, because you start with those who are already ill (prevalence cases), you cannot calculate an incidence (new cases) rate. However, you can still calculate an approximation of the relative risk, which is the **odds ratio (OR)**: an estimate of the risk of *being* sick, not *becoming* sick (Kahn & Sempos, 1989).

Let's go back to your study of the 10 patients with the unknown disease causing respiratory failure. In addition to your sample of 10 sick patients, you select 10 healthy controls from the community. After completing your interviews and chart reviews, you see that 6 of the sick patients recently traveled to Eastern Asia and lived in villages where wild birds were raised among the community. Two others worked in a chicken processing plant. Four of your healthy controls also had some type of bird exposure but were not sick. You decide to calculate an OR to see what association may be found between the illness and exposure to some type of bird. You set up another 2 × 2 table. See Figure 12-2.

Figure 12-2 Exposure to Birds and Respiratory Failure.

	Cases	Controls	Total
Exposure	A = 8	B = 4	12
No exposure	C = 2	D = 6	8
Total	10	10	20

Because this is a case control study, you calculate an OR that divides the odds that a case was exposed by the odds that a control was exposed. Odds and probability are two different things. Odds are the chances that something happens divided by the chance that it doesn't. For example, if the probability of your passing an exam is 80%, the chance that you won't is 20%. The odds of your passing the exam are 80% ÷ 20%, or 4:1 (Gordis, 2000).

To calculate the odds of a case being exposed using the 2 × 2 table, divide *A* by *C*. In the example, this would be 8 ÷ 2; in plain English, the odds that a sick patient was exposed to birds are 4:1. The odds of a control being exposed are *B* ÷ *D*, or 4 ÷ 6, or 0.66. To get the odds ratio, take 4 ÷ 0.66 to get 6.06. The odds are six times higher that a case (sick patient) was exposed to the birds than a healthy control. You can do a bit of math and determine that the equation can actually be simplified to

$$\frac{AD}{BC}$$

In this example:

$$\frac{8 \times 6}{4 \times 2} = 6$$

If you find that version easier, you are welcome to do it. If you hate to memorize things (as I do), think about what the OR means and figure out the math from there.

You will see OR and RR used more frequently in the public health and nursing literature because they make for easier understanding by the general public. If you are using the OR to estimate the RR, you can then report that your study *estimates* that individuals exposed to the birds are six times as likely to be sick or that exposure to the birds is associated with an estimated six-fold increase in risk of developing this illness. If these results are significant, they can help the investigator determine the possible causative agent for the respiratory failure by

prompting funding for a cohort study or for further investigation. They can also be used to convey public health concerns to the public in a readily understandable way.

When using the OR to estimate the RR, the researcher should be aware that the results are the most accurate when the cases are rare (< 10% incidence or prevalence) and the cases and controls should be representative of the population in terms of the exposure of interest (Sullivan, 2008). Also, OR is an estimate of the RR, not the same thing; so if you are using this tool incorrectly, your results may not be meaningful.

Cross-Sectional Study

The last type of study frequently used in epidemiology literature is a **cross-sectional study**, which collects the data about exposure and outcome at the same time. For example, suppose you surveyed the nurses on your unit and asked them how many hours they worked that day and if they were tired. You would have data, but not a time sequence. The data is all collected at the same time. This is a significant limiting factor because you cannot determine the direction of the relationship even if you find one. For example, in your survey about work hours and fatigue, you might hypothesize that the hours a nurse works is associated with fatigue. However, with a cross-sectional survey, you cannot assume that the hours worked came before the fatigue. What if the nurse actually came to work fatigued because her spouse is out of work and she deals with a lot of stress at home. She may still work an extra shift that is requested because she needs the additional income, but her fatigue actually started before she came to work. You don't know whether the fatigue is related to the hours worked or to preexisting factors or to factors that contributed to the decision to work extra hours. Cross-sectional studies offer preliminary results and can be useful in forming hypotheses, but they are usually only the beginning of the examination of any significant research issue.

Attributable Risk

Attributable risk is another concept that makes sense to most nonstatisticians and therefore is a helpful tool when you are disseminating public health information. **Attributable risk for the exposed group** (AR_e) tells you the amount of a disease or outcome in an exposed group that is due to a particular exposure. It is very easy to calculate. The formula is:

$$AR_e = \text{Incidence rate in the exposed group} - \text{Incidence rate in the nonexposed group}$$

For example, let's say you develop a cohort study to examine the relationship between tanning bed usage and cataract development. You put your results in the 2 × 2 table shown in Figure 12-3. The incidence rate for the exposed group is 60 per 100. The incidence rate for the unexposed group is 10 per 100. (This is what is considered background risk, or the risk for everyone who does not have the exposure you are looking at.) The attributable risk for the exposed group

is the difference: $60/100 - 10/100 = 50/100$, or 50 cases per 100 individuals. If tanning beds were eliminated, you could prevent up to 50 cases of cataracts for 100 individuals who would have tanned before this new policy. (Of course, they could just slather on the baby oil and hit the beaches; this is why you can only say *up to* 50 cases.)

To make this number meaningful, determine the proportion of the excess risk (beyond background risk) that is associated with exposure to tanning beds by dividing 50 by 60 (the incidence in the exposed group): 0.83, or 83%. This tells you how much of the risk of cataracts is due to tanning beds *in those who used the tanning beds.*

How could you use this information clinically? You might advise your patients who tan that, if they stop using the tanning beds, they could reduce their risk of developing cataracts by 83%. That is information that most patients will understand much more easily than if you start talking about incidence and relative risk (Gordis, 2000).

It is also the type of information that large populations can understand and that is meaningful to public officials, not to mention making a great headline!

Figure 12-3 Tanning Bed Exposure and Cataract Development.

	Cataracts	No cataracts	Totals
Tanning bed usage	60	40	100 (exposed)
No tanning	10	90	100 (nonexposed)
Totals	70 (diseased)	130 (nondiseased)	200

Summary

You have now completed Chapter 12 and should be feeling very confident with this material. To review some key concepts, let's start with epidemiology.

Epidemiology is the study of the distribution of disease. Three types of epidemiological studies are the cohort study, case control study, and cross-sectional study.

A cohort study is done by following a group of individuals over time to see who develops the outcome of interest. Remember to exclude prevalence cases in this design because they already have the trait you are studying or wish to study. The incidence data you collect allows you to determine the number of new cases among your sample during the duration of your study. The relative risk is the incidence rate in the exposed sample divided by the incidence rate of those not exposed.

A protective effect occurs anytime you have a significant relative risk less than one. A relative risk of one means that there is no association between the exposure and the illness. An exposure is considered an associated risk factor for the disease when the relative risk is greater than one and the p-value is significant.

A case control study involves starting with the outcome of interest and working backward to determine exposure. The odds ratio is used to calculate the approximation of the relative risk. You must have incidence data to calculate a relative risk. The odds ratio uses prevalence data (those who are already sick).

In a cross-sectional design, you collect data about exposure and outcomes at the same time.

Public health information has to be delivered in a way that the general public can understand. The attributable risk in the exposed group converts research results into meaningful information for the media and for the general public. People need to be able to understand the important clinical information you have worked so hard to determine!

These new concepts will be helpful to you in mastering statistics, particularly if you are interested in becoming an epidemiologist (a blatant plug for epidemiology).

CHAPTER 12 REVIEW QUESTIONS

Questions 1–9: The variables in Figure 12-4 have been examined to determine the association with a length of labor.

Figure 12-4 Variables Related to Length of Labor > 12 Hours.

Variable	RR	95% CI	*p*-value
Maternal age < 40			
Yes	0.87	(0.72–1.23)	0.23
No (reference group)	1.00		
Support person present			
Yes	0.43	(0.31–0.56)	0.03
No (reference group)	1.00		
Previous birth			
Yes	0.21	(0.18–0.24)	0.01
No (reference group)	1.00		
Epidural anesthesia			
Yes	1.20	(1.06–1.34)	0.02
No anesthesia or IV/IM anesthesia (reference group)	1.00		

1. What are your "exposure" or independent variables?

   _____

   _____

2. What is your outcome or dependent variable?

   _____

3. If you instead measure your dependent variable rounded to the nearest full hour, what level of measurement is it? Is it quantitative or qualitative?

   _____

(continues)

4. Suppose you originally measured this variable as a yes-or-no response to the question, "Did you feel as though you had a very long labor?" What level of measurement was it? Was it a quantitative or qualitative question?

_____

_____

5. If the study has an alpha of 0.05, which variables are associated with the length of labor? Which are associated with a decreased length of labor? Which are associated with an increased length of labor?

_____

_____

_____

6. Note that when the *p*-value is significant, the RR confidence intervals do not include the value of one. Why?

_____

7. Did maternal age significantly increase the risk of having a labor > 12 hours?

_____

8. Did using epidural anesthesia significantly increase the risk of having a longer labor? Compared to whom?

_____

9. Interpret in English the RR for maternal age and length of labor.

_____

_____

10. A study reports that children who have breakfast are more likely to pass the fourth-grade math competency ($RR = 1.39, 95\% \, CL = 1.30 - 1.49$). You know that, because the 95% confidence limits do not include an RR of 1, these results are:

_____

Questions 11–15: The sleep disorder clinic conducted a small cohort study with medical residents working 24 hour shifts to examine how exposure to caffeine, melatonin, strenuous exercise, or television affects the risk of medical residents falling asleep 2 hours later. The results are shown in Figure 12-5.

Figure 12-5 Factors Related to Risk of Falling Asleep 2 Hours After Exposure.

Variable	RR	95% CI
Caffeine	0.67	0.55–0.75
Melatonin	1.34	1.21–1.46
Exercise	0.88	0.70–1.18
Television	0.93	0.89–0.99

11. What factors are significantly related to the risk of the residents falling asleep?

12. What is the dependent or outcome variable?

13. Which exposure had the greatest impact on the risk of falling asleep 2 hours after exposure?

14. Interpret the RR for television. Is it significant?

15. Which exposure was most effective in decreasing the risk of falling asleep 2 hours later?

Questions 16–17: The study was replicated, but this time the researchers examined the effect of these exposures on sleep 6 hours later. See Figure 12-6.

Figure 12-6 Factors Related to Risk of Falling Asleep 6 Hours After Exposure.

Variable	RR	95% CI
Caffeine	0.89	0.54–1.51
Melatonin	1.02	0.80–1.45
Exercise	1.34	1.17–2.08
Television	0.96	0.89–0.99

(continues)

16. Offer a reasonable explanation for this.

_____

_____

17. A taxi company wants to implement a policy to diminish the risk of falling asleep behind the wheel. The company has the greatest number of accidents due to drivers falling asleep on the evening shift between 9 and 11 p.m. They are considering either opening the company gym for use by the cab drivers between 1 and 3 p.m. or making free coffee available during the dinner hour (6–7 p.m.). Which policy would this research support implementing?

_____

Questions 18–20: A cohort study following a group of 200 randomly selected adolescent males find the results shown in Figure 12-7.

18. Calculate the incidence rate for traumatic injury.

_____

19. What is the attributable risk for the exposed group? Interpret the risk in English.

_____

20. Calculate the RR of traumatic injury for adolescent males who consume alcohol. Assuming your RR is significant, interpret this value.

_____

Figure 12-7 Alcohol Use and Traumatic Injury in Adolescent Males.

	Traumatic injury	No traumatic injury	Totals
Alcohol use	98	40	138
No alcohol use	10	52	62
Totals	108	92	200

Use your computer to practice these applications.

The companion website for this book has a computer-based application example for this material. Check it out!

Analyze	Graphs	Utilities	Add-ons	Window	Help

Reports ▶

Descriptive Statistics ▶   📊 Frequencies...

Tables ▶   📊 Descriptives...

Compare Means ▶   🔍 Explore...

General Linear Model ▶

Generalized Linear Models ▶   🔲 Crosstabs...

ANSWERS TO CHAPTER 12 REVIEW QUESTIONS

1. Maternal age < 40, having a support person present, previous births, and epidural anesthesia

3. Interval, quantitative

5. Having a support person present (decreased risk of labor > 12 hours), having had previous births (decreased risk of labor > 12 hours), and using epidural anesthesia (increased risk of labor > 12 hours)

7. No, RR is not significant

9. Answers will vary. For example, Maternal age less than 40 years is not significantly associated with the risk of labor > 12 hours.

11. Caffeine, melatonin, television

13. Melatonin increased falling asleep 2 hours later.

15. Caffeine

17. Free coffee! Exercise 6 hours before going on shift would increase the number of time the cab drivers fell asleep, whereas coffee 2 hours before the shift would decrease it.

19. $98 \div 138 - 10 \div 62 = 0.71 - 0.16 = 55\%$: Fifty-five out of 100 of the cases of injuries in adolescent men are in adolescents who consume alcohol.

References

Agresti, A. (2002). *Categorical data analysis* (2nd ed.). Wiley Series in Probability and Statistics. Hoboken, NJ: Wiley.

Anifantaki, S., Prinianakis, G., Vitsaksaki, E., Katsouli, V., Mari, S., Symianakis, A., et al. (2009). Daily interruption of sedative infusions in an adult medical-surgical intensive care unit: Randomized control trial. *Journal of Advanced Nursing*, 65(5), 1054–1060.

Chen, M., Shiao, Y., & Gau, Y. (2007). Comparison of adolescent health-related behavior in different family structures. *Journal of Nursing Research*, 15(1), 1–10.

Chung, Y.C., & Hwang, H. L. (2008). Education for homecare patients with with leukemia following a cycle of chemotherapy: An exploratory pilot study [online exclusive]. *Oncology Nursing Forum*, 35(5), E86–E87.

Cohen, J. (1988). *Statistical power analysis for the behavioral sciences* (2nd ed.) Hillsdale, NJ: Lawrence Erlbaum Associates.

Corless, I., Lindgren, T., Holzemer, W., Robinson, L., Moezzi, S., Kirksey, K., et al. (2009). Marijuana effectiveness as an HIV self-care strategy. *Clinical Nursing Research*, 18(2), 172–193.

Corty, E. W. (2007). *Using and interpreting statistics: A practical text for the health, behavioral and social sciences.* St. Louis, MO: Mosby.

Doering, L., Cross, R., Magsarili, M., Howitt, L., & Cowan, M. (2007). Utility of observer-rated and self-report instruments for detecting major depression in women after cardiac surgery. *American Journal of Critical Care*, 16(3), 260–269.

Fallovollita, J., Luisi, A. J., Jr., Michalek, S. M., Valverde, A. M., deKemp, R. A., Haka, M. S., et al. (2006). Prediction of arrhythmic events with positron emission tomography. *Contemporary Clinical Trials*, 27(4), 374–388.

Fowler, J., Jarvis, P., & Chevannes, M. (2002). *Practical statistics for nursing and health care.* West Sussex, UK: John Wiley & Sons.

Gordis, L. (2002). *Epidemiology* (2nd ed.). Philadelphia, Penn.: W. B. Saunders.

Grove, S. K. (2007). *Statistics for health care research: A practical workbook.* St. Louis, MO: W. B. Saunders.

Heyman, H., Van De Looversosch, D., Jeijer, E., & Schols, J. (2008). Benefits of an oral nutritional supplement on pressure ulcer healing in long-term care. *Journal of Wound Care, 17*(11), 476–480.

Johnson, N. L., & Kotz, S. (1997). *Leading personalities in statistical sciences.* Wiley Series in Probability and Statistics: Probability and Statistics Section. Hoboken, NJ: Wiley.

Kahn, H., & Sempos, C. (1989). *Statistical methods in epidemiology.* New York: Oxford University Press.

Munro, B. H. (2005). *Statistical methods for health care research* (5th ed.). Philadelphia: Lippincott Williams & Wilkins.

New York State Nurses Association. (n.d.). *Mandatory overtime law.* Retrieved August 3, 2010, from http://www.nysna.org/practice/mot/intro.htm

Nieswiadomy, R. (2008). *Foundations of nursing research* (5th ed.). Upper Saddle River, NJ: Pearson Education.

Norman, G. R., & Streiner, D. L. (2008). *Biostatistics: The bare essentials* (3rd ed.). Hamilton, ON: BC Decker Inc.

Oepkes, D., Seaward, P. G., Vandenbussche, F. P., Windrim, R., Kingdom, J., et al. (2006). Doppler ultrasonography versus amniocentesis to predict fetal anemia. *New England Journal of Medicine, 355*(2), 156–164.

Olbrys, K M. (2001). The effect of topical lidocaine anesthetic on reported pain in women who undergo needle wire localization prior to breast biopsy. *Southern Online Journal of Nursing Research, 6*(2), 1–18.

Pagano, M., & Gauvreau, K. (1993). *Principles of biostatistics.* Belmont, CA: Wadsworth.

Papastavrou, E., Tsangari, H., Kalokerinou, A., Papacostas, S., & Sourtzi, P. (2009). Gender issues in caring for demented relatives. *Health Science Journal, 3*(1), 41–53.

Plichta, S. B., & Garzon, L. S. (2009). *Statistics for nursing and allied health.* Philadelphia: Wolters Kluwer Health/Lippincott Williams & Wilkins.

Schilling, F., Spix, C., Berthold, F., Erttmann, R., Fehse, N., et al. (2002). Neuroblastoma screening at one year of age. *New England Journal of Medicine, 346*(14), 1047–1053.

Sullivan, L. M. (2008). *Essentials of biostatistics in public health.* Sudbury, MA: Jones and Bartlett.

Szklo, M., & Nieto, F.J. (2000). *Epidemiology: Beyond the basics.* Gaithersburg, MD: Aspen Publishers.

Tobian, A., Serwadda, D., Quinn, T. C., Kigozi, G., Gravitt, P. E., et al. (2009). Male circumcision for the prevention of HSV2 and HPV infection and syphilis. *New England Journal of Medicine, 360*(13), 1298–1309.

Vassiliadou, A., Stamatopoulou, E., Triantafyllou, G., Gerodimou, E., Toulia, G., & Pistolas, D. (2008). The role of nurses in the sexual counseling of patients after myocardial infarction. *Health Science Journal, 2*(2), 111–118.

Watson, R., Atkinson, I., & Egerton, P. (2006). *Successful statistics for nursing & healthcare.* Hampshire, UK: Palgrave Macmillan.

Zellner, K., Boerst, C., & Tabb, W. (2007). Statistics used in current nursing research. *Journal of Nursing Education, 46*(2), 55–59.

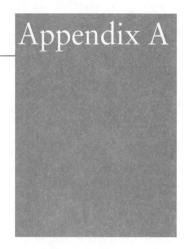

Practice Article: Doering et al.

Using what you know.

The following exercise gives you the opportunity to synthesize what you have learned and to see how statistics is used in actual nursing research. First, read the full text of the article, and then start to work your way through the questions that follow. As you start to dissect each portion of the article, you should go back to the article and also into your text for reference and refresh your mind. Your answers may not exactly match the answers given. The answers given are to be used as a reference so that you can check yourself. If you don't understand some of them, make sure you go back and review the relevant portion of the article and your text. This is a great way to review for a cumulative final and also a really good way to help yourself retain the information you worked so hard to master.

The articles in the appendices are set up to focus on different concepts, all the while supporting and enhancing the knowledge you have mastered in each of the chapters.

Happy reading!

Utility of Observer-Rated and Self-Report Instruments for Detecting Major Depression in Women After Cardiac Surgery: A Pilot Study

By Lynn V. Doering, RN, DNSc, Rebecca Cross, RN, MSN, FNP, Marise C. Magsarili, RN, MN, Loretta Y. Howitt, MD, and Marie J. Cowan, RN, PhD

Background Major depression is common after coronary artery bypass graft surgery and is associated with increased mortality and morbidity. Clinicians have few practical options for detecting depression, especially in women, who are at higher risk for depression than men.

Objectives To evaluate the clinical utility of common self-report and observer-rated instruments for detection of major depression in women after coronary artery bypass graft surgery.

Methods In 66 women being discharged after coronary artery bypass graft surgery, 4 instruments were completed: the Hamilton Depression Rating Scale, Beck Depression Inventory, Beck Depression Inventory Short Form, and Beck Depression Inventory for Primary Care. For each instrument, receiver-operating characteristic curves were analyzed, and positive and negative predictive values were calculated for cutoff points determined from the curves.

Results At hospital discharge, all 4 instruments yielded highly accurate curves. Compared with cutoffs suggested for patients without medical illness and hospitalized nonsurgical patients, identified cutoffs for screening were higher when all types of depressive symptoms (cognitive, affective, behavioral, somatic) were measured with the Hamilton Depression Rating Scale and the Beck Depression Inventory but lower when only cognitive and/or affective symptoms were measured with the 2 subscales of the Beck Depression Inventory.

Conclusions The Hamilton Depression Rating Scale and both subscales of the Beck Depression Inventory may be useful for detecting major depression in women shortly after coronary artery bypass graft surgery. Further study is warranted to confirm cutoffs in these patients. (American Journal of Critical Care. 2007;16: 260-269)

About the Authors Lynn V. Doering is an associate professor, Rebecca Cross is a doctoral candidate, and Marie J. Cowan is a professor and dean in the University of California–Los Angeles School of Nursing. Marise C. Magsarili is a nurse practitioner and Loretta Y. Howitt is a physician with Kaiser Permanente Medical Center in Los Angeles, Calif.

Corresponding author: Lynn Doering, RN, DNSc, FAAN, UCLA School of Nursing, 700 Tiverton Ave, Factor 4-266, Los Angeles, CA 90095-6918 (e-mail: ldoering@sonnet.ucla.edu).

In adults with coronary artery disease, depression is common and dangerous.[1,2] Adults undergoing coronary artery bypass graft (CABG) surgery are particularly susceptible; signs and symptoms of depression are extremely common both before and after surgery.[3-5]

Prevalence reports range from 32% to 65% for signs and symptoms within 1 week before surgery and from 20% to 46% for signs and symptoms measured up to 6 months after surgery.[6] Clinical depression after CABG surgery has rarely been described; 17% to 20% of patients have postoperative major depression, and an additional 27% of patients have minor depression.[7,8] In contrast, the 12-month prevalence of major depression in community samples of adults is 5.5% to 10.8%.[9,10] With approximately 306000 patients undergoing CABG surgery annually in the United States,[11] approximately 61000 of them are likely to experience major depression. Depressed patients, compared with nondepressed patients, have a higher rate of depression-related mortality and morbidity after CABG surgery, more cardiac events and postoperative complications such as hospital readmissions, and higher healthcare costs.[7,12-14]

In general, rates of depression in women are higher than the rates in men, and outcomes in women tend to be worse.[15] Although few reports address depression in women after CABG surgery, rates of depression in women with ischemic heart disease and women with heart failure follow this general pattern. Among patients with heart failure, women are more likely to be depressed than men, and depressed patients tend to be younger than nondepressed patients.[16]

In the Enhancing Recovery in Coronary Heart Disease trial, female patients reported higher levels of depression and distress than did male patients; the greatest differences occurred among younger women.[17] In women undergoing CABG surgery, depression occurs at rates similar to the rates in women with heart failure and the rates in other clinical populations, such as women with diabetes.[18,19] Compared with men, women may be particularly susceptible to depression after CABG surgery because women tend to become depressed after a triggering event, such as surgery.[20]

Despite the prevalence of depression after CABG surgery and its association with mortality and morbidity, clinicians have few practical options for detecting depression, especially in women. Structured diagnostic interviews, such as the Diagnostic Interview and Structured Hamilton (DISH) or the Structured Clinical Interview for the *Diagnostic and Statistical Manual, Fourth Edition (DSM-IV)*, are well validated and reliable but require extensive training and are time-consuming to administer.[21,22] Alternatively, self-report and observer instruments have the advantage of being short and easier to use than structured interviews, but most were designed to measure the severity of signs and symptoms of depression only rather than clinical depression.

Among self-report instruments, the Beck Depression Inventory (BDI) is considered the reference standard.[23] Although it was originally developed for use in psychiatric patients, the BDI has been widely used in both healthy and medically ill populations. Recently, new subscales of the BDI for use with medically ill patients have been developed, including a 13-item version of all cognitive/affective items in the BDI, called the BDI Short Form (BDI-SF),[24] and a 7-item version of selected cognitive/affective items, called the BDI for Primary Care (BDI-PC).[25] Among observer-rated instruments, the Hamilton Depression Rating Scale (HDRS) is the most widely accepted.[26] Like the BDI, the HDRS has been used widely in medically ill populations.

Beck's cognitive model of depression offers an appropriate theoretical framework for evaluating these instruments.[27] Beck postulates that depressed individuals have a negative bias in their view of themselves, their world, and their future. This negative bias is evident in their cognitive function, in the form of automatic thoughts and negative core schema. Negative cognitive bias triggers negative affective, somatic, and behavioral responses. Thus, evaluation of cognitive, affective, somatic, and behavioral symptoms merit consideration in detecting clinical depression. This theory is consistent with the *DSM-IV* criteria, the HDRS, and the BDI, all of which include all of these elements; differences exist in the type and number of characteristics assessed in each. By contrast, the BDI-SF and the BDI-PC include only cognitive and/or affective items.

Because clinicians have little information to guide evaluation of depression in women during the period shortly after CABG surgery, the purpose of this pilot study was to evaluate the clinical utility of self-report and observer-rated instruments for detecting depression in this population. The specific aims of the study were to determine the sensitivity and specificity of the 2 instruments that included all categories of depressive symptoms (HDRS and BDI) and of 2 instruments that included only cognitive and/or affective symptoms (BDI-SF and BDI-PC) for detection of major depression in women before hospital discharge after CABG surgery.

Methods

Design

The investigation reported here was conducted as part of a pilot study to test the effects of nurse-administered home cognitive behavioral therapy in women with major depression after CABG surgery. For this report, a cross-sectional design was used in which women were evaluated for major depression by using a diagnostic interview at the time of hospital discharge after CABG surgery, and the presence or absence of depression was correlated with depression scores on self-reported and observer-rated instruments.

Sample and Setting

Women were recruited from 2 tertiary care centers in a major metropolitan area. After the study was approved by institutional review boards, women were invited to participate if they were no more than 75 years old, were having CABG surgery for the first time, and spoke English. A convenience sample of 66 women who completed the predischarge diagnostic evaluation, the observer rating interview, and the BDI as part of the parent study was used.

Procedures

Before each patient was discharged from the hospital, informed consent was obtained, and a research nurse administered the Mini-Mental Status Examination. After confirming a score of 24 or greater on that examination, which is consistent with a lack of cognitive impairment,[28,29] a trained interviewer (L.V.D.) administered the DISH before the patient was discharged from the hospital. To confirm the diagnostic results of the interview, all patients classified as depressed were evaluated by a psychiatrist. After both interviews, participants completed the BDI with instructions to consider how they had been feeling for the past 2 weeks. Research assistants who administered the BDI had no knowledge of the results of the diagnostic interview.

Instruments

DIAGNOSTIC INTERVIEW AND STRUCTURED HAMILTON

The DISH is a semi-structured interview designed to form of automatic thoughts and negative core schema. Negative cognitive bias triggers negative affective, somatic, and behavioral responses. Thus, evaluation of cognitive, affective, somatic, and behavioral symptoms merit consideration in detecting clinical depression. This theory is consistent with the *DSM-IV* criteria, the HDRS, and the BDI, all of which include all of these elements; differences exist in the type and number of characteristics assessed in each. By contrast, the BDI-SF and the BDI-PC include only cognitive and/or affective items.

Because clinicians have little information to guide evaluation of depression in women during the period shortly after CABG surgery, the purpose of this pilot study was to evaluate the clinical utility of self-report diagnose depression in medically ill patients.[21] In validation studies, the DISH and Structured Clinical Interview for *DSM-IV* resulted in 88% agreement (κ = .86).[21] Interrater reliability has been established, with 93% agreement between diagnosis by trained interviewers and clinicians and with diagnostic agreement across symptom clusters (κ = .75).[21,30]

BECK DEPRESSION INVENTORY

The BDI is a 21-item self-reported measure of the intensity of signs and symptoms of depression, with items rated 0 to 3 (0 = no signs or symptoms, 3 = most severe signs and symptoms) and totals ranging from 0 to 63. Suggested guidelines for cutoff scores are less than 10 for no or minimal depression, 10 to 18 for mild to moderate depression, 19 to 28 for moderate to severe depression, and 29 and higher for severe depression. The BDI is used routinely to monitor changes in signs and symptoms in cognitive behavioral therapy. Concurrent validity of the BDI has been supported by correlations between the BDI and selected concurrent measures of depression and by agreement with clinical psychiatric evaluations of

depression.[31] Meta-analyses of internal consistency have yielded Cronbach α coefficients of .86 for psychiatric patients and .81 for nonpsychiatric patients.[32]

Among CABG patients, internal consistency of the BDI is high, with Cronbach α coefficients of .82.[33] Widely used to assess the severity of depression in psychiatric patients, the BDI also has been validated in older adults[34] and across a variety of medical populations, including patients with diabetes[35] or chronic pain[36] and patients undergoing hemodialysis.[37] The BDI has demonstrated utility for differentiating among medical, nonmedical, and healthy groups[32] and is a sensitive indicator of cardiac mortality.[38] It has shown discriminative validity in distinguishing higher from lower sympathetic nervous activation in women tested for severity of depressive symptoms.[39] In the study reported here, tests of internal consistency yielded a Cronbach α coefficient of .92.

BECK DEPRESSION INVENTORY SHORT FORM

The BDI-SF includes all 13 cognitive/affective items in the BDI. The BDI-SF was developed in response to concerns that in medically ill populations the use of somatic items to evaluate depressive symptoms might lead to spuriously high scores and overreporting of depression.[23] As with the BDI, items are scored from 0 (no signs or symptoms) to 3 (most severe signs and symptoms); total scores range from 0 to 39. The use of only the cognitive/affective items was suggested to assess depression in medically ill patients, with the use of scores of 10 or greater as a cutoff for moderate to severe depressive syndromes.[24] With this cutoff, the BDI-SF has demonstrated high sensitivity (100%) and negative predictive value (100%) in patients hospitalized in a general medical ward.[24] With a cutoff of 8 or greater, the BDI-SF had adequate sensitivity (79%) and negative predictive value

(96%) with diagnostic interviews in a sample of terminally ill cancer patients receiving palliative care and was well correlated ($r = 0.96$) with the original 21-item scale.[40] In the study reported here, tests of internal consistency yielded a Cronbach α coefficient of .89.

BECK DEPRESSION INVENTORY FOR PRIMARY CARE

Like the BDI-SF, the BDI-PC was designed to minimize the possibility of yielding spuriously high estimates of depression in patients with medical illnesses by focusing on cognitive/affective signs and symptoms. For the BDI-PC, 7 items were selected purposefully to correspond to *DSM-IV* criteria (sadness and anhedonia), to capture important clinical indicators of risk in depressed patients (suicidality), and to reflect those items that loaded most saliently ($\geq$ .35) on the cognitive dimension of the original instrument (pessimism, past failure, self-dislike, and lack of confidence).[41] As with the BDI and BDI-SF, the items are scored from 0 to 3 to reflect intensity of the sign or symptom, but the BDI-PC includes only 7 items. Totals range from 0 to 21. A cutoff of 4 and higher yields strong sensitivity (82%-83%) and specificity (82%-95%) rates for detection of major depression in medical inpatients and outpatients.[25,42] In the study reported here, tests of internal consistency yielded a Cronbach α coefficient of .87.

HAMILTON DEPRESSION RATING SCALE

The 17-item version of the HDRS is administered via a structured interview in which subjects are asked to respond to questions about the signs and symptoms they had during a specific (2-week) period. Responses are rated by the interviewer, with 8 affective/cognitive items rated on a 5-point scale (0 = no signs or symptoms, 4 = most severe signs and symptoms) and 9 somatic items rated on a 3-point scale (0 = no signs or symptoms, 2 =

most severe signs and symptoms). Scores range from 0 to 52. Scores of 24 or higher are generally agreed to indicate severe depression, whereas scores of 18 to 23 represent the moderate range, 7 to 17 signify mild depression, and scores less than 7 indicate no depression.[26] The HDRS is sensitive to change over time and treatment and agrees well with overall clinical ratings of severity.[43] It has well-documented validity, with a Cronbach α of .81 recently reported[44]; recent studies also support interrater reliability, with intraclass correlations of 0.96 to 0.97.[45,46] For this study, administration time for the HDRS was approximately 30 minutes.

Analysis

Measures of central tendency and dispersion were used to describe the sample. For comparing depressed with nondepressed patients, a *t* test was used for continuous variables and a χ^2 test for categorical variables. For each of the instruments and subscales (HDRS, BDI, BDI-SF, and BDI-PC), receiver-operating-characteristic (ROC) curves were analyzed to generate plots of sensitivity versus 1 minus specificity for detecting major depression for every possible cutoff point and to generate graphs of the area under the curve (AUC). The AUC is equivalent to the probability that a randomly selected individual from the positive reference sample has a greater test value than a randomly selected individual from the negative reference sample; an appropriate sample estimate is made by using the nonparametric Mann-Whitney *U* test.[47] Curves are ranked against noninformative curves as less accurate (0.5 < AUC < 0.7), moderately accurate (0.7 < AUC < 0.9), highly accurate (0.9 < AUC < 1.0), and perfect (AUC = 1.0).[47]

Standard formulas were used to calculate positive and negative predictive value for cutoff points determined from each curve. To focus on the utility of instruments for both screening (detecting depressive symptoms) and diagnosis (detecting cases of major depression), we examined each curve for cutoff points that would maximize sensitivity and negative predictive value (for screening) and specificity and positive predictive value (for diagnosis).

Results

[Characteristics of the sample as a whole and by depression status at hospital discharge are presented in Table 2.] At hospital discharge, 7 women (11%) met the diagnostic criteria for major depression; of these, 4 had a history of depression ($P = .06$). Compared with women without depression, depressed women were less educated ($P = .01$). Preoperative risk did not differ significantly between groups. During hospitalization, the rates of complications, including incidence of perioperative myocardial infarction and acute renal failure, were similar in depressed and nondepressed women. Women with major depression at discharge had experienced longer periods of postoperative intubation than had women without depression (28.6% vs 5.2%, $P = .03$). Regarding medical treatment at hospital discharge, the administration of aspirin, β-blockers, statins, and hormone replacement therapy did not differ significantly between groups.

For the whole sample, median scores for the HDRS, BDI, BDI-SF, and BDI-PC were 8, 8, 2, and 1, respectively. Interquartile ranges (25%-75%) for the instruments were 3 to 13.25, 3 to 13, 0 to 5.5, and 0 to 3, respectively. For the HDRS, 55.4% of patients scored at or above the usually accepted cutoff for nonmedically ill patients of 7. For the BDI, 43.9% scored 10 or higher, the recommended cutoff for depressive symptoms in nonmedically ill patients. For the BDI-SF and the BDI-PC, 20% and 23.1% scored above the cutoffs of 8/9 and

4, respectively, recommended for medically ill patients.[24,41] With all 4 instruments, scores of depressed and nondepressed patients differed significantly.

The Figure presents the ROC curve analyses for detection of major depression at hospital discharge. All 4 instruments yielded strong ROC curves, with AUCs exceeding .900 considered highly accurate.[47] Cutoff points derived from each curve were examined for sensitivity, specificity, positive predictive value, and negative predictive value. For each instrument, cutoffs from these data differed from those reported in the literature. For the HDRS and BDI, cutoffs for both screening (HDRS ≥ 14, BDI ≥ 12) and diagnosis (HDRS ≥ 19, BDI ≥ 24) were higher than those usually reported for symptom onset (HDRS ≥ 7, BDI ≥ 10). For the cognitive/affective-only instruments (BDI-SF and the BDI-PC), we found lower cutoffs for screening (BDI-SF ≥ 4, BDI-PC ≥ 2) than previously reported (BDI-SF ≥ 8, BDI-PC ≥ 4). Similarly, diagnostic cutoffs for these instruments (BDI-SF ≥ 12, BDI-PC ≥ 5) were lower than those previously reported (BDI-SF ≥ 13, BDI-PC ≥ 6).

Discussion

To our knowledge, this is the first study in which the BDI and its shorter cognitive-based forms, along with the HDRS, were evaluated concurrently in medically ill patients. At the time of patients' discharge from the hospital after CABG surgery, all 4 instruments yielded ROC curves consistent with highly accurate tests, with AUCs exceeding .900. These data provide important albeit initial support for the utility of all 4 instruments as tests for major depression at the time of hospital discharge after CABG surgery. Although these data are encouraging, further analysis in larger studies is needed to confirm these findings.

Evaluation of HDRS and BDI

For screening, on the basis of the ROC curves at hospital discharge, we were able to identify cut-offs with high sensitivity (100%) and negative predictive value for each instrument. According to the evaluation of misclassified cases, the HDRS yielded the fewest false-positives and indicated all true cases. A cutoff of 14 or greater (higher than the standard cutoff of 7 or greater) on the HDRS may be reasonable for depression screening in women after CABG surgery. In a recent evaluation[48] of the BDI for screening patients with myocardial infarction 1 month after the index infarction, an optimal screening cutoff of 7 or greater was reported when both major and minor depression were considered. The higher cutoff of 12 or greater that we observed for screening with the BDI is probably due to our focus on major depression only.

Evaluation of Cognitive-Only Instruments

According to Beck's theory, instruments used to measure all types of signs and symptoms of depression (cognitive, affective, somatic, and behavioral) should be more accurate for detecting major depression than are instruments used to measure only cognitive/affective signs and symptoms. In the evaluation of medically ill patients, both clinicians and researchers have continued to debate the merits of including somatic signs and symptoms as part of clinical depression.[49-51] For screening of adults hospitalized in medical wards for at least 72 hours, Furlanetto et al[24] found that a BDI-SF cutoff of 9 or greater produced the highest sensitivity and negative predictive value.

In our study, the designated cutoff of 4 or greater also allowed detection of all cases of depression. In both studies, the false-positive rates were high, with many nondepressed patients identified as depressed by means of the BDI-SF. For diagnosis, we again observed a somewhat lower cutoff (≥ 12) than that observed in hospitalized medical patients (≥ 14). The discrepancy between the cutoff we identified and those in the earlier report may be due to the different study populations. Compared with general medical patients, surgical patients about to be discharged from the hospital may have had blunting of affective signs and symptoms of depression, as indicated by the low medians and interquartile ranges that we observed. In our surgical population, the median BDI-SF score in nondepressed patients was 2, and 25% of depressed patients scored as low as 6. Thus, compared with the cutoff for patients with medical problems, a relatively low cutoff was required for our surgical patients to ensure high sensitivity for screening and high specificity for diagnosis.

In 2 earlier reports,[52,53] the BDI-SF was only moderately accurate in patients hospitalized with diverse medical problems, with an AUC of .85 to .87. Nonetheless, in these reports, the recommended cutoff of 4 or higher produced relatively high sensitivities of 90% to 91%. Again, the optimal cutoffs we observed were lower than those previously recommended. As with the BDI-SF, we suspect that the characteristics of depressive signs and symptoms in patients after CABG surgery must differ in some way from the signs and symptoms of the previously studied medical patients.

When all 4 instruments are considered, patients who have had CABG surgery seem to require a higher threshold for both screening and diagnosis when multimodal instruments (HDRS and BDI) are used, whereas lower thresholds are required when cognitive/affective-only instruments (BDI-SF and BDIPC) are used. Although further study is needed to confirm these findings, the presence of postoperatively generated somatic signs and symptoms may explain the higher thresholds for the HDRS and the BDI.

Conversely, in the case of the BDI-SF and BDIPC, the omission of somatic signs and symptoms may yield a greater influence of cognitive/affective signs and symptoms, so that a lower level of cognitive/affective signs and symptoms is associated with clinical depression.

Study Limitations

Our study had several limitations. First, we studied only women, so our findings are not generalizable to men or to mixed samples of men and women. Second, our sample size was small. Determination of sample size for ROC analysis depends on interobserver accuracy, accuracy of the curves (AUC), and the ratio of positive and negative cases.[54] The adequacy of our sample is supported by our use of a single observer to make all diagnostic determinations (thus eliminating interobserver error), the generation of ROC curves with high accuracy at hospital discharge, and the finding of a prevalence of major depression at hospital discharge similar to the prevalence reported in other studies[48] of cardiac patients. Therefore, our sample size should have been sufficient for detecting cases of depression at hospital discharge.

In addition, some differences (eg, a history of clinical depression) between depressed and nondepressed patients might not have been identified because the sample size was small and thus vulnerable to type II error. However, further studies with larger samples that include a greater proportion of depressed women and men would be important to confirm these findings and enhance generalizability across diverse samples of CABG surgery patients. Likewise, further refinement of cutoff points and testing for relevance against different sociodemographic strata in CABG surgery patients would be valuable.

Clinical Significance

Although these pilot data should be used cautiously in drawing inferences for clinical practice, they are clinically significant for testing. For screening, an ideal instrument would have high sensitivity and negative predictive value so that the chance of missing true cases of major depression would be minimized. Thus, all truly depressed patients would be recognized and would receive more in-depth evaluation to confirm the diagnosis. If the purpose of testing is to streamline diagnosis of major depression and enhance recognition of true cases, then high specificity and positive predictive value would be more important.

For example, the HDRS is an observer-rated instrument that requires the rater to assess patients' responses to specific items. Therefore, the HDRS requires more time and training than does the BDI. For settings in which clinicians' training and time limit the use of the HDRS, the BDI or its 2 shorter cognitive forms may be reasonable alternatives. These self-report instruments usually take less than 10 minutes to complete, and all yielded somewhat more false-positives than the HDRS, but still indicated all true cases with the screening cutoff given {in Table 3}. Of note, cutoff associated with all instruments differed from those standard accepted cutoffs. Further testing in larger samples is warranted to confirm these findings and further evaluate appropriate cutoffs for screening and diagnosis.

Conclusion

These findings provide initial support for the use of both observer (HDRS) and self-report (BDI, BDI-SF, BDI-PC) instruments to test for depression in women at hospital discharge after CABG surgery. For the clinical purposes of testing (screening or diagnoses), cutoffs higher than usually recommended for medically ill patients should be considered when instruments including a variety of depressive symptoms (such as the

HDRS and the BDI) are used. When instruments that include only cognitive/affective symptoms (such as the BDI-SF and BDI-PC) are used, lower cutoffs may be more helpful for both screening and diagnosis. Further study in larger samples of patients who have undergone CABG surgery is warranted.

Financial Disclosures This study was supported by grants NIMH K01MH01700 and R01NR009228 from the National Institute of Mental Health.

References

1. Carney RM, Freedland KE. Depression, mortality, and medical morbidity in patients with coronary heart disease. Biol Psychiatry. 2003;54:241-247.

2. Frasure-Smith N, Lesperance F. Depression and other psychological risks following myocardial infarction. *Arch Gen Psychiatry*. 2003;60:627-636.

3. Burker EJ, Blumenthal JA, Feldman M, et al. Depression in male and female patients undergoing cardiac surgery. *Br J Clin Psychol*. 1995; 34:119-128.

4. McKhann GM, Borowicz LM, Goldsborough MA, Enger C, Selnes OA. Depression and cognitive decline after coronary artery bypass grafting. *Lancet*. 1997;349:1282-1284.

5. Pirraglia P, Peterson J, Williams-Russok P, Gorkin L, Charlson M. Depressive symptomatology in coronary artery bypass graft surgery patients. *Int J Geriatr Psychiatry*. 1999;14:668-680.

6. McCrone S, Lenz E,Tarzian A, Perkins S. Anxiety and depression: incidence and patterns in patients after coronary artery bypass graft surgery. *Appl Nurs Res*. 2001;14:155-164.

7. Connerney I, Shapiro PA, McLaughlin JS, Bagiella E, Sloan RP. Relation between depression after coronary artery bypass surgery and 12-month outcome: a prospective study. *Lancet*. 2001;358: 1766-1771.

8. Doering L, Gerard I, Magsarili M, Cowan M. Women after cardiac surgery: more than just the blues [abstract]. *Circulation*. 2002;106:II-539.

9. Kessler RC, McGonagle KA, Zhao S, et al. Lifetime and 12month prevalence of DSM-III-R psychiatric disorders in the United States: results from the National Comorbidity Survey. *Arch Gen Psychiatry*. 1994;51:8-19.

10. Dunlop DD, Song J, Lyons JS, Manheim LM, Chang RW. Racial/ethnic differences in rates of depression among preretirement adults. *Am J Public Health*. 2003;93:1945-1952.

11. American Heart Association. *Heart Disease and Stroke Statistics: 2005 Update*. Dallas,Tex: American Heart Association; 2005.

12. Baker RA, Andrew MU, Schrader G, Knight JL. Preoperative depression and mortality in coronary artery bypass surgery: preliminary findings. *ANZ J Surg*. 2001;71:139-142.

13. Saur CD, Granger BB, Mulbaier LH, et al. Depressive symptoms and outcome of coronary artery bypass grafting. *Am J Crit Care*. 2001; 10:4-10.

14. Scheier MF, Matthews KA, Owens JF, et al. Optimism and rehospitalization after coronary artery bypass graft surgery. *Arch Intern Med*. 1999;159:829-835.

15. Kessler RC, Berglund P, Demler O, et al.The epidemiology of major depressive disorder: results from the National Comorbidity Survey Replication (NCS-R). *JAMA*. 2003;289:3095-3105.

16. Gottlieb SS, Khatta M, Friedmann E, et al.The influence of age, gender, and race on the prevalence of depression in heart failure patients. *J Am Coll Cardiol*. 2004;43:1542-1549.

17. Mendes de Leon C, Dilillo V, Czajkowski S, et al. Psychosocial characteristics after acute myocardial infarction: the ENRICHD pilot study. Enhancing Recovery in Coronary Heart Disease. *J Cardiopulm Rehabil*. 2001;21:353-362.

18. Anderson RJ, Freedland KE, Clouse RE, Lustman PJ. The prevalence of comorbid depression in adults with diabetes: a meta-analysis. *Diabetes Care*. 2001;24:1069-1078.

19. Freedland KE, Rich MW, Skala JA, et al. Prevalence of depression in hospitalized patients with congestive heart failure. *Psychosom Med*. 2003;65:119-128.

20. Carandang JM, Franco-Bronson K, Kamarei S. Recognizing and managing depression in women throughout the stages of life. *Cleve Clin J Med*. 2000;67:329-331.

21. Freedland KE, Skala JA, Carney RM, et al. The Depression Interview and Structured Hamilton (DISH): rationale, development, characteristics, and clinical validity. *Psychosom Med*. 2002;64:897-905.

22. Miller PR, Dasher R, Collins R, Griffiths P, Brown F. Inpatient diagnostic assessments, I: accuracy of structured vs unstructured interviews. *Psychiatry Res*. 2001;105:255-264.

23. Richter P, Werner J, Heerlein A, Kraus A, Sauer H. On the validity of the Beck Depression Inventory: a review. *Psychopathology*. 1998;31:160-168.

24. Furlanetto LM, Mendlowicz MV, Romildo Bueno J. The validity of the Beck Depression Inventory-Short Form as a screening and diagnostic instrument for moderate and severe depression in medical inpatients. *J Affect Dis*. 2005;86:87-91.

25. Steer RA, Cavalieri TA, Leonard DM, Beck AT. Use of the Beck Depression Inventory for primary care to screen for major depression disorders. *Gen Hosp Psychiatry*. 1999;21:106-111.

26. Endicott J, Cohen J, Nee J, Fleiss J, Sarantakos S. Hamilton Depression Rating Scale: extracted from regular and change versions of the schedule for affective disorders and schizophrenia. *Arch Gen Psychiatry*. 1981;38:98-103.

27. Beck AT. The current state of cognitive therapy: a 40-year retrospective. *Arch Gen Psychiatry*. 2005;62:953-959.

28. Tombaugh TN, McIntyre NJ. The Mini-Mental State Examination: a comprehensive review. *J Am Geriatr Soc*. 1992;40:922-935.

29. Joray S, Wietlisbach V, Bula CJ. Cognitive impairment in elderly medical inpatients: detection and associated six-month outcomes. *Am J Geriatr Psychiatry*. 2004;12:639-647.

30. Miller GE, Freedland KE, Carney RM, Stetler CA, Banks WA. Pathways linking depression, adiposity, and inflammatory markers in healthy young adults. *Brain Behav Immun*. 2003;17:276-285.

31. Beck A, Steer R. *Beck Depression Inventory Manual*. San Antonio, Tex: Psychological Corp; 1987.

32. Beck A, Steer R. Psychometric properties of the Beck Depression Inventory: twenty-five years of evaluation. *Clin Psychol Rev*. 1988;8:77-100.

33. Artinian N, Duggan C. Sex differences in patient recovery patterns after coronary artery bypass surgery. *Heart Lung*. 1995;24:483-494.

34. Gallagher D, Nies G, Thompson L. Reliability of the Beck Depression Inventory with older adults. *J Consult Clin Psychol*. 1982;50:152-153.

35. Sullivan B. Adjustment in diabetic adolescent girls, II: adjustment, self-esteem, and depression in diabetic adolescent girls. *Psychosom Med*. 1979; 41:127-138.

36. Turner J, Romano J. Self-report screening measures for depression in chronic pain patients. *J Clin Psychol*. 1984;40:909-913.

37. Rhodes L. Social climate perception and depression of patients and staff in a chronic hemodialysis unit. *J Nerv Ment Dis*. 1981;169:169-175.

38. Frasure-Smith N, Lesperance F, Juneau M, Talajic M, Bourassa MG. Gender, depression,

and one-year prognosis after myocardial infarction. *Psychosom Med.* 1999;61:26-37.

39. Light K, Kothandapani R, Allen M. Enhanced cardiovascular and catecholamine responses in women with depressive symptoms. *Int J Psychophysiol.* 1998;28:157-166.

40. Chochinov HM, Wilson KG, Enns M, Lander S. "Are you depressed?" Screening for depression in the terminally ill. *Am J Psychiatry.* 1997;154:674-676.

41. Beck AT, Guth D, Steer RA, Ball R. Screening for major depression disorders in medical inpatients with the Beck Depression Inventory for Primary Care. *Behav ResTher.* 1997;35:785-791.

42. Beck A, Steer R, Ball R, Ciervo C, Kabat M. Use of the Beck Anxiety and Beck Depression Inventories for Primary Care with medical outpatients. *Assessment.* 1997;4:211-219.

43. Cicchetti D, Prusoff B. Reliability of depression and associated clinical symptoms. *Arch Gen Psychiatry.* 1983;40:987-990.

44. Bent-Hansen J, Lunde M, Klysner R, et al. The validity of the depression rating scales in discriminating between citalopram and placebo in depression recurrence in the maintenance therapy of elderly unipolar patients with major depression. *Pharmacopsychiatry.* 2003;36:313-316.

45. Zimmerman M, Posternak M, Chelminski I. Is the cutoff to define remission on the Hamilton Rating Scale for Depression too high? *J Nerv Ment Dis.* 2005;193:170-175.

46. DeRubeis RJ, Hollon SD, Amsterdam JD, et al. Cognitive therapy vs medications in the treatment of moderate to severe depression. *Arch Gen Psychiatry.* 2005;62:409-416.

47. Greiner M, Pfeiffer D, Smith RD. Principles and practical application of the receiver-operating characteristic analysis for diagnostic tests. *Prev Vet Med.* 2000;45:23-41.

48. Strik JJ, Honig A, Lousberg R, Denollet J. Sensitivity and specificity of observer and self-report questionnaires in major and minor depression following myocardial infarction. *Psychosomatics.* 2001;42:423-428.

49. Leetjens A, Verhey F, Luijckx G, Troost J. The validity of the Beck Depression Inventory as a screening and diagnostic instrument for depression in patients with Parkinson's disease. *Move Disord.* 2000;15:1221-1224.

50. Lustman J, Clouse R, Griffith L, Carney R, Freedland K. Screening for depression in diabetes using the Beck Depression Inventory. *Psychosom Med.* 1997;59:559-560.

51. Lykouras L, Oulis P, Adrachta D, et al. Beck Depression Inventory in the detection of depression among neurological inpatients. *Psychopathology.* 1998;31:213-219.

52. Wilhelm K, Kotze B, Waterhouse M, Hadzi-Pavlovic D, Parker G. Screening for depression in the medically ill: a comparison of self-report measures, clinician judgment, and DSMIV diagnoses. *Psychosomatics.* 2004;45:461-469.

53. Parker G, Hilton T, Bains J, Hadzi-Pavlovic D. Cognitive-based measures screening for depression in the medically ill: the DMI-10 and the DMI-18. *Acta Psychiatr Scand.* 2002;105:419-426.

54. Obuchowski NA. Sample size tables for receiver operating characteristic studies. *AJR Am J Roentgenol.* 2000; 175:603-608.

APPENDIX A REVIEW QUESTIONS

1. Begin with the abstract (summary) of the article. What was the purpose of the study?

_____

_____

2. Why is this an important clinical issue?

_____

_____

At this point you already know what the study is trying to do and why it matters. Great start! Now let's dive into the article itself. Usually, research articles begin with a literature review that establishes what the research already tells us and why the study is being done. Let's see what role statistics can play in this portion of a research article.

3. The authors begin by stating that "in adults with coronary artery disease (CAD) depression is common and dangerous." How do the authors support this statement using statistics? What do these statistics mean?

_____

_____

4. If depression after CABG surgery were a benign condition, it might not be important to detect. For example, if the presence of depression was associated only with the type of toothpaste you selected the next day, the toothpaste company might want to fund the study, but the National Institute of Health probably would not. Therefore, to strengthen the argument that depression in women after CABG surgery is an important issue to address, the nurse researchers need to support that the outcomes associated with the presence of depression are significant. How is statistics used to do this?

_____

_____

5. Now the authors go on to use statistics in another way. They already told us there are few measures of depression in women after CABG surgery, but there are reports of rates in a "similar population": those with coronary heart disease or heart failure. Do they report a difference in the gender-specific prevalence rates of depression in these women?

_____

_____

6. The researchers then present information about the measurement tools they wish to examine in this study. They already have a valid and reliable tool, the structured diagnostic interview, to detect depression. What do we know about this tool from this description?

_____

_____

7. Why not just keep using this tool if we already know it works?

_____

_____

8. What are the advantages and disadvantages of the self-report and observer instruments used to detect depression?

_____

_____

9. What test is the so-called gold standard (the one that will be used to establish that depression exists and to test whether the other measures are able to detect it)?

_____

_____

10. Now let's look at the actual design of the study. What type of study design was utilized?

_____

_____

11. What sampling technique was used?

_____

_____

12. What concerns do you have about the sampling technique?

_____

_____

13. What is the target population for this study, and for whom can you generalize the results?

_____

_____

(continues)

14. What is the sample size? Assuming the standard alpha of 0.05 and power of 0.80, do you anticipate they will have the power to detect a large or small effect size?

_____

_____

15. With the small sample size, what type of error would be most concerning, and what would be the result?

_____

_____

16. Now let's look at the actual measures used in the study and the statistics behind them. The researchers report that the structured diagnostic interview using DISH has an inter-rater reliability of 93%. What does this mean about the instrument?

_____

_____

17. The nurse researchers report that the Beck Depression Inventory (BDI) has items rated on a scale of 0 to 3 with 0 being no signs or symptoms and 3 being the most severe. Is each item categorical or continuous? Is the total score a continuous or categorical measure?

_____

_____

18. What level of measurement are the individual items in the BDI? What would be the most appropriate measure of central tendency for these items?

_____

_____

19. What level of measurement is the total score on the BDI?

_____

_____

20. What options do researchers have for calculating a measure of central tendency for the BDI total score?

_____

_____

21. The nurse researchers report that concurrent validity (which is another name for convergent validity) is established for the BDI. What does this tell you?

_____

_____

22. The researchers go on to say that the Cronbach alpha coefficient is 0.92 in this study. What does this mean?

_____

_____

23. The study also talks about a modification of the BDI [Beck Depression Inventory to develop the Beck Depression Inventory Short-Form (BDI-SF)]. The BDI-SF was developed because of concerns that the original BDI, which included physical signs and symptoms of depression, might overdiagnose depression if used with populations who are medically ill. (This is a perfect example of being careful not to overgeneralize results.) The appropriate total score in a medically healthy population indicating depression may not be appropriate for a population that has medical illnesses contributing additional physical symptoms. The modified BDI-SF was designed for detecting depression in medically ill patients. When using a cutoff of a score of 10, the BDI-SF has a sensitivity of 100% and a negative predictive value of 100% for hospitalized patients. What does this mean?

_____

_____

24. In another study, the total score on the BDI-SF was found to be well correlated ($r = 0.96$) with the total score on the original BDI. What does this mean?

_____

_____

25. The BDI was also modified and shortened for use in a primary care setting (BDI-PC). The specificity of the BDI-PC is 82–95% for detecting major depression in medically ill populations. What does this mean?

_____

_____

(continues)

26. Now that you've dissected some of the measurement issues, let's look at the analysis portion of the article. In this section, the nurse researchers explain how they analyzed the information they gathered in the structured interview (DISH) and the self-reported and observer-related tools administered when the patients were discharged post-CABG. The authors begin by explaining that they compared the measures of central tendency and dispersion for two groups: (1) those who were depressed (determined by the gold standard DISH interview and psychiatric evaluation) and (2) those who were nondepressed. They used a t-test for continuous variables and a chi-square test for categorical variables.

    One of the variables used for comparison was educational level. What would be an appropriate null hypothesis for this comparison? What would be an appropriate alternative hypothesis?

    _____

    _____

27. Suppose educational level is measured as, "Did not graduate from high school" and "Graduated from high school." What level of measurement is this variable?

    _____

    _____

28. What statistical test would you use to test your hypothesis, and why? The resulting p-value is 0.01. What does this mean? If during your analysis you realize that one of the cells in your 2×2 table had only four subjects, which test would you use?

    _____

    _____

29. The nurse researchers then used several statistical techniques that were beyond the scope of this book to determine the best cutoff points (scores on the tests) for the different measurement tools for screening and diagnosis of depression. Refer to the FTS in Chapter 4, and explain why the cutoff for screening focuses on maximizing sensitivity and negative predictive value, whereas the cutoff for diagnosis maximizes specificity and positive predictive value.

    _____

    _____

30. Now let's look at the results section, which explains what all the statistical testing produced. What was the prevalence rate for depression?

_____

_____

31. Was there a statistically significant difference in educational level for the subjects who were depressed and those who were not?

_____

_____

32. Was there a statistically significant difference in preoperative risk between the two groups?

_____

_____

33. Was there a difference in the postoperative intubation time for the two groups?

_____

_____

34. What was the median score for the original BDI in the whole sample, and what does this mean?

_____

_____

35. What was the interquartile range for the whole sample on the original BDI, and what does that mean?

_____

_____

36. If you use the cutoff of a score of 10 on the BDI to diagnose depression, what percentage of patients meet the diagnostic criteria?

_____

_____

(continues)

37. Which measurement tools detected significant differences between the patients who were depressed and those that were not?

_____

_____

38. The researchers examined the mean age of the patients who were depressed and those who were not. Write appropriate null and alternative hypotheses. What would be a good statistical test for this analysis, and why? The corresponding *p*-value is 0.25. What do you conclude?

_____

_____

39. The study concludes that all four of the observer-related or self-reported instruments have value in detecting depression in women post-CABG at the time of discharge. They each have a lower cutoff score for screening than for diagnosis. The sensitivity and negative predictive value of all the instruments for screening is 100%. Why is this information clinically relevant?

_____

_____

40. Based on this article, if you need to screen a patient from a similar target population for depression at hospital discharge post-CABG, what measurement instrument should you use?

_____

_____

ANSWERS TO APPENDIX A REVIEW QUESTIONS

1. To evaluate the clinical utility of common self-report and observer-rated instruments for the detection of major depression in women after coronary artery bypass graft (CABG) surgery

3. Prevalence reports tell you how many cases there are in a population at any given time and give you a measure of the disease burden in the population. The authors compare prevalence rates in the population of adults who undergo CABG to those in the general community and report much higher percentages in the population of individuals who have CABG. This means the disease burden in the population of individuals who undergo CABG surgery is much higher than in the general population.

   They also apply prevalence rates to the total number of individuals who undergo CABG surgery annually in the United States to estimate the total number of cases of major depression within this group. This gives an absolute measure of the number of individuals who may be affected rather than a percentage or rate. This may help some readers grasp the enormity of the problem.

   They also report higher rates of poor outcomes in this group, although these rates are not quantified.

5. Yes, women have higher rates, particularly younger women. Although not quantified, the authors use gender- and age-specific rates to identify the population at greatest risk.

7. It is long and has to be administered by a person with extensive training. This requirement also increases the cost (educational training and the cost for the time it takes the person to administer the interview and the patient to complete it).

9. The gold standard test is the structured diagnostic interview by a trained interviewer (for example, the DISH). In this study, those who were classified as depressed also had the diagnosis confirmed by a psychiatrist.

11. Nonprobability sampling. A convenience sample was collected from two tertiary care centers in a metropolitan area.

13. The target population is defined by the inclusion criteria. Participants must be women under 75 years old who are having their first CABG surgery and who speak English. The generalizability of the study is limited to this population. For example, you should not take the rates of depression detected in this group and then apply them to men.

15. A type two error would miss a difference that really exists between the measurement instruments.

(continues)

17. Each item is a categorical variable.

    The total score is continuous and can be converted into categorical results using the suggested cutoffs.

19. Ratio

21. The BDI and other measures of depression, such as clinical evaluations, consistently indicate the same results, thereby supporting the validity(accuracy) of the measurement instrument.

23. One hundred percent sensitivity means that all the patients who had the disease (depression) when measured by a gold standard tested positive for the disease when they were given the BDI-SF. (They all scored 10 points or more.)

    One hundred percent negative predictive value means that, of the subjects who tested negative (scored less than 10 points on the BDI-SF), all of them did not have the disease.

25. Specificity rates of 82–95% mean that, of those subjects who really are well, 82–95% will screen/test negative with the BDI-PC. In other words, 82–95% of those who are healthy will score below four points on the BDI-PC and not be diagnosed with depression.

27. Ordinal

29. A sensitive screen is very good at identifying subjects who are actually sick, and high negative predictive value means you can be pretty sure those who test negative are not sick. (Start with the big fishing net or the low-resolution lens to narrow the sample down to those who are more likely to be sick and confidently eliminate those who test negative.) Then, for diagnosis, specificity and positive predictive value become more important. High specificity and positive predictive value increase your confidence in a positive result, meaning those who test positive are likely to be positive. (You switch to high power on the microscope and narrow the sample down to only those who are really sick, becoming more confident in the positive test results.)

31. Yes, $p = 0.01$

33. Yes, women with major depression at discharge had longer periods of postoperative intubation, $p = 0.03$.

35. When you consecutively line up the BDI scores for the whole sample, the middle 50 percent fall between a score of 3 and a score of 13.

37. All four: HDRS, BDI, BDI-SF, and BDI-PC

39. You know that all four screens do not miss true cases.

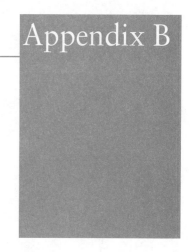

Practice Article: Chang et al.

Using what you know.

This appendix presents another opportunity for you to use what you have learned in the course to better understand an actual nursing research article. Read through the following article by Drs. Chang, Wang, and Chao, and answer the questions after the text. You will again find that statistics plays a part throughout the study and that you now understand a great deal more from the article than you would have before you took the course. Enjoy!

Influence of Physical Restraint on Unplanned Extubation of Adult Intensive Care Patients: A Case-Control Study

By Li-Yin Chang, RN, MSN, Kai-Wei Katherine Wang, RN, PhD, and Yann-Fen Chao, RN, PhD

Background Unplanned extubation commonly occurs in intensive care units. Various physical restraints have been used to prevent patients from removing their endotracheal tubes. However, physical restraint not only does not consistently prevent injury but also may be a safety hazard to patients.

Objectives To evaluate the effect of physical restraint on unplanned extubation in adult intensive care patients.

Methods A total of 100 patients with unplanned extubations and 200 age-, sex-, and diagnosis-matched controls with no record of unplanned extubation were included in this case-control study. The 300 participants were selected from a population of 1455 patients receiving mechanical ventilation during a 21-month period in an adult intensive care unit at a medical center in Taiwan. Data were collected by reviewing medical records and incident reports of unplanned extubation.

Results The incidence rate of unplanned extubation was 8.7%. Factors associated with increased risk for unplanned extubation included use of physical restraints (increased risk, 3.11 times), nosocomial infection (increased risk, 2.02 times), and a score of 9 or greater on the Glasgow Coma Scale on admission to the unit (increased risk, 1.98 times). Episodes of unplanned extubation also were associated with longer stays in the unit.

Conclusions An impaired level of consciousness on admission to the intensive care unit and the presence of nosocomial infection intensify the risk for unplanned extubation, even when physical restraints are used. To minimize the risk of unplanned extubation, nurses must establish better standards for using restraints. (*American Journal of Critical Care.* 2008; 17:408-416)

About the Authors Li-Yin Chang is supervisor of the nursing department at Taichung Veterans General Hospital and is a doctoral student in the School of Nursing, National Yang-Ming University, Taipei, Taiwan. Kai-Wei Katherine Wang is an assistant professor in the School of Nursing at National Yang-Ming University, Taipei, Taiwan. Yann-Fen Chao is a professor in the College of Nursing at Taipei Medical University, Taipei, Taiwan.

Corresponding author: Yann-Fen Chao, RN, PhD, College of Nursing, Taipei Medical University, 250 Wu-Xin St, Taipei City, Taiwan 110 (e-mail: yfchao.tw@yahoo.com.tw).

Unplanned extubation is common in intensive care units (ICUs). For most patients, removal of the endotracheal tube and weaning from mechanical ventilation are planned by the medical team. However, some patients deliberately remove the endotracheal tube when they are irritable or uncomfortable, or it may be accidentally removed while a patient is being transported or during a nursing intervention.[1] The reported incidence rate of unplanned extubation in intensive care patients ranges from 3.4%[2] to 22.5%.[3] In the past, various restraints have been used to prevent unplanned extubation as well as falls and injuries. Physical restraints include any device, material, or equipment that is attached to a person's body and deliberately prevents the person's free bodily movement. However, the reported incidences of unplanned extubation, even when physical restraints are used, have not changed appreciably in recent years.[4] Furthermore, several studies[5] have shown that physical restraint not only does not consistently prevent injury, but may increase the possibility of injury and become a safety hazard to patients.

Literature Review

Risk factors associated with unplanned extubation include both patient- and nursing-related factors. Risk factors related to patients include restlessness, agitation, confusion, physical suffering, nosocomial infection, and oral (vs nasotracheal) intubation.[1,4,6] Risk factors related to nursing include poor fixation of the endotracheal tube,[7] high patient-to-nurse ratios, and the night shift.[3,8]

Unplanned extubation of patients who require mechanical ventilation can be life-threatening; the most serious consequences are cardiopulmonary arrest and death.[2] The reported reintubation rates after unplanned extubation are 36%

to 57% for the first hour[9-11] and 37% to 57% within 48 hours.[3,6,12,13] Replacement of the endotracheal tube often can lead to hemodynamic and airway complications.[14] Unplanned extubation and reintubation are associated with longer total duration of mechanical ventilation, ICU stay, and hospital stay.[6,12] Prevention of unplanned extubation remains an important issue in critical care.

Problems with unplanned extubation in ICUs can be handled with or without restraints. Some investigators[15,16] have suggested that restraining an unconscious or restless patient might prevent selfextubation, whereas other researchers[17] are concerned that use of restraints might cause anxiety and increase the possibility of unplanned extubation. Nevertheless, self-extubation occurs despite the use of sedation and restraints. The reported percentage of unplanned extubations initiated by restrained patients varies widely, from 25.6% to 80%.[1,3,18]

Sedation, a chemical form of restraint, has been proposed to decrease the incidence of unplanned extubation. However, sedation increases the risk for unplanned extubation by prolonging mechanical ventilation and initiating paradoxical agitation.[4] Physical restraints remain the first choice when unplanned extubation is considered a high risk. The inconsistent effect of physical restraints on preventing unplanned extubation[15-17] is confusing for clinicians. Evidence is required to guide the decision about whether or not to use physical or chemical restraints to decrease unplanned extubation.

Purpose

The relationship between unplanned extubation and physical restraints may differ in various settings. We conducted this retrospective study to analyze risk factors and explore the influence of physical restraints on unplanned extubation. The aims of the study were to (1) identify the factors associated with increased risk for unplanned extubation and (2) determine the risk factors for unplanned extubation in patients with and without physical restraints.

Methods

Design and Sample

This retrospective, case-controlled study was conducted in a 42-bed, open-room setting, adult ICU at Taichung Veterans General Hospital, Taichung, Taiwan, Republic of China. The mean number of years that nursing staff had worked in the ICU was 4.85 (SD, 3.73; range, 2-19). The study population included all patients who were admitted and intubated in this adult ICU during a 21-month period (between October 2003 and July 2005). The unplanned extubation group consisted of 100 patients receiving mechanical ventilation who had an unplanned extubation; the control group consisted of 200 patients receiving mechanical ventilation who had no record of unplanned extubation.

In order to increase the statistical power of the study, 2 control patients were selected for each patient who had an unplanned extubation.[19] Case matching was based on each patient's age, sex, diagnosis, and dates of hospital stay. The incidence rate of unplanned extubation was calculated as follows: [(total number of patients with unplanned extubation)/(total number of intubated patients)] × 100. The incidence density of unplanned extubation was calculated as [(total number of patients with unplanned extubation)/(total number of days of mechanical ventilation)] × 100.

The unplanned extubation group had better GCS scores on admission, more nosocomial infections, and higher use of physical restraints.

Data Collection

Data were collected by reviewing medical records and incident reports of unplanned extubations and completing a structured data collection sheet. Data included patients' demographics, admission diagnosis, score on the Acute Physiological and Chronic Health Evaluation (APACHE) II, total length of ICU/hospital stay, and the following data related to the unplanned extubation: consciousness status, days of mechanical ventilation, ventilation parameters, presence of nosocomial infection, use of sedation, and use of physical restraint. The information on nosocomial infection was offered by the infection control committee and was based on the standard of the Centers for Disease Control and Prevention.[20] In this study, sedatives were drugs used to modify behavior, including hypnotic agents (propofol or etomidate) and nondepolarizing muscle relaxants.

Ethical Considerations

The study was approved by the ethical review board of the hospital. The standard protocol for physical restraint in this unit was (1) an evaluation of the risk of unplanned extubation and/or fall, with a physician explaining the necessity of physical restraint to the patient and the patient's family; (2) after obtaining the written medical order and getting the informed consent form signed by the patient or the patient's family member, the nurse restraining the patient with a proper device; (3) at 2-hour intervals, the nurse removing the physical restraint, performing a massage and range-of-motion exercises on the restrained joints, and documenting observations of the restrained area.

Data Analysis

Data were analyzed by using SPSS software (version 12.0 for PC, SPSS Inc, Chicago, Illinois). The major statistical procedures used in this study were χ^2 test, risk estimation, Mann-Whitney test, t test, receiver-operating-characteristic curve analysis, and logistic regression. A power analysis based on the effect size of the data indicated that the sample size had a power greater than 90% at the significance level of .05 for the χ^2 test, t test, and regression analysis.

Results

Incidence Rate of Unplanned Extubation

In a 21-month period, 126 episodes of unplanned extubation occurred in 1455 patients receiving mechanical ventilation. The incidence rate of unplanned extubation was 8.7% and the incidence density of unplanned extubation was 2.07%. Patients in the unplanned extubation group had diagnoses of pneumonia (37.5%), chronic obstructive pulmonary disease (21.5%), substance intoxication (14%), and cancer (6%). The mean duration of mechanical ventilation before unplanned extubation was 8.6 days (SD, 7.4); 14% of such extubations occurred on the first day, 54% within the first 7 days, and 79% within the first 14 days. The mean score on the Glasgow Coma Scale (GCS) at the time of unplanned extubation was 10.6 (SD, 0.8).

A total of 68 patients were reintubated. The main reason for reintubation was respiratory distress (63 patients). The remaining 5 patients were reintubated because of poor cough ability. Among the 68 patients, 55 were reintubated within 1 hour. From the 126 patients who had an unplanned extubation, we selected the 100 patients who had their first and only unplanned extubation and finished their ICU stay during our study period as the unplanned extubation group. A total of 200 patients from the same population matched for age, sex, diagnosis, and duration of

ICU stay who had no record of unplanned extubation were used as the control group.

[The characteristics of the unplanned extubation and control groups are listed in Table 1.] The mean APACHE II scores were 21.2 (SD, 7.5; range, 3-63) for the unplanned extubation group and 22.4 (SD, 7.3; range, 6-44) for the control group. No significant differences were apparent in age, sex, APACHE II scores, route of intubation, and sedative status between the 2 groups. The unplanned extubation group had better GCS scores on admission (mean [SD], 10.1 [2.2] vs 9.2 [3.0], $P = .002$), higher rates of nosocomial infection (26.0% vs 12.5%, $P = .004$), and higher rates of use of physical restraint (82.0% vs 54.5%, $P < .001$). The types of nosocomial infection did not differ significantly in frequency between groups ($P = .29$). The unplanned extubation group also had a longer ICU stay than did the control group (mean [SD], 22.9 [16.4] vs 16.5 [13.3], $P = .001$).

Use of Physical Restraint

Among the total of 300 patients, 191 were physically restrained during their ICU stay. In an effort to identify the factors contributing to and the consequences of use of physical restraints, characteristics were compared between patients who were physically restrained and patients who were not [Table 2]. The 2 groups did not differ significantly in age, sex, APACHE II score, days of intubation, route of intubation, or sedative status. The physical restraint group had better GCS scores on admission (mean [SD], 10.0 [2.3] vs 8.6 [3.3], $P < .001$) and higher rates of nosocomial infection (21.5% vs 9.2%, $P = .005$) than the other group. The physical restraint group had higher rates of unplanned extubation (42.9% vs 16.5%, $P < .001$) and longer ICU stay (mean [SD], 20.3 [15.1] days vs 15.8 [13.5] days; $P = .009$) than the other group.

Risk Factors for Unplanned Extubation

Among the 191 patients who were physically restrained, 82 had an unplanned extubation. Background information was compared between patients in the unplanned extubation group and patients in the control group to identify the factors contributing to unplanned extubation [Table 3, upper section]. Age, APACHE II scores, GCS score, restraint method, route of intubation, and sedative status did not differ significantly between the unplanned extubation and control groups. However, the unplanned extubation group had a higher rate of nosocomial infection than did the control group (29.3% vs 15.6%, $P = .02$).

Among the 109 subjects who were never physically restrained during their ICU stay, 18 had an unplanned extubation. Background information was compared between patients in the unplanned extubation group and patients in the control group in an effort to identify factors contributing to unplanned extubation if the subjects were not physically restrained [Table 3, lower section]. Although the unplanned extubation group and the control group had no significant differences in age, APACHE II scores, route of intubation, rates of nosocomial infection, or sedative status, the unplanned extubation group had higher GCS scores on ICU admission than did the control group (mean [SD], 10.3 [2.2] vs 8.3 [3.4], $P = .004$).

Multivariate Risk Estimate of Unplanned Extubation

A forward logistic regression model was used to examine the summative risk of the occurrence of unplanned extubation. The variable selected first was physical restraint, next was presence of nosocomial infection, and the last was GCS score on ICU admission. A receiver-operating-characteristic curve procedure was applied to examine the best cutoff point of the GCS score for predicting unplanned extubation. A GCS score of 9 had a sensitivity of 85.0% and a specificity of 80.8%. Physical restraint, presence of nosocomial infection, and GCS score of 9 were entered in a logistic regression procedure again; [the results are summarized in Table 4]. The overall accuracy rate of this model was 69%. From the model, the relative risk of a patient with a GCS score of 9 for an unplanned extubation was 1.98. If physical restraint was used on such a patient, the risk of unplanned extubation increased to 6.16 (1.98 $\times$ 3.11). If the presence of nosocomial infection was added, then the risk of unplanned extubation increased to 12.44 (1.98 $\times$ 3.11 $\times$ 2.02). The cumulative risk of various combination situations is illustrated in the Figure.

Discussion

Incidence Rate and Factors Associated with Increased Risk of Unplanned Extubation

The incidence rate of unplanned extubation in our study was 8.7%, which was higher than that in the study by Pandey et al[2] (3.4%) and lower than that in the study by Yeh et al[3] (22.5%). The 350 ventilator-dependent ICU patients enrolled in the study by Pandey et al[2] had been receiving mechanical ventilation for 48 hours or more. As a result, unplanned extubations on the first 2 days after intubation were not included. In our study, 41% of unplanned extubations happened within 48 hours after intubation. This difference between the studies may account for the lower incidence rate for unplanned extubation reported by Pandey et al.[2] In the study by Yeh et al,[3] a total of 1176 ICU patients were enrolled from

11 ICUs where 39.2% of the nurses had less than 2 years of work experience. In our study, all the nurses had worked in the ICU for more than 2 years. Another explanation for the high incidence rate for unplanned extubation in the study by Yeh et al is that the unplanned extubation occurred most often when inexperienced nurses were caring for patients.

In our study, the mean duration of intubation before unplanned extubation was 8.6 (SD, 7.4) days, and 54% of unplanned extubations occurred in the first 7 days. These findings are similar to that in the study by Pesiri et al,[15] in which 60% of unplanned extubations occurred within 7 days of intubation.

We matched the unplanned extubation group and the control group by age, sex, diagnosis, and duration of hospitalization; no significant difference in these variables was expected. The APACHE II scores of the 2 groups were similar. Therefore, the severity of patients' conditions had similar effects on the results in the 2 groups. However, the unplanned extubation group had significantly better GCS scores, as well as higher rates of use of physical restraint and nosocomial infection, than did the control group [Table 1]. These 3 variables (level of consciousness, use of physical restraints, and development of infection) were also significant predictors of unplanned extubation according to multivariate logistic regression [Table 4].

Influence of Physical Restraints on Patients Who Had Unplanned Extubation

In this study, 82% of unplanned extubations occurred in patients with physical restraints. This finding is similar to the results of other studies,[1,3] which indicate that use of physical restraint not only is inadequate in preventing unplanned extubation but actually promotes unplanned extubation. Because the GCS scores

and rates of nosocomial infection were higher in physically restrained subjects [Table 2], it seems likely that patients who had a higher level of consciousness and also had a nosocomial infection had higher rates of being physically restrained, and the 3 risk factors tended to aggregate and led to unplanned extubation. However, GCS scores did not differ significantly between the unplanned extubation group and the control group if the patients were physically restrained, and infection rates did not differ significantly between the unplanned extubation group and the control group if the subjects were not physically restrained [Table 3]. These results indicate that physically restrained patients with nosocomial infection and patients with better neurological status who are not physically restrained are most at risk for unplanned extubation. In other words, the risk of unplanned extubation can be due to the use of physical restraints and the presence of nosocomial infection.

Similarly, the risk of unplanned extubation is greater when the patient is not under physical restraint and the patient's GCS score on ICU admission is 9 or greater. Patients with better GCS scores are more responsive to sensory stimuli. This greater responsiveness may explain the increased risk of unplanned extubation in patients with GCS scores of 9 or more. Therefore, physical restraint should be applied only when it is essential to a patient's safety or chemical restraint (sedative therapy) is not appropriate. When such a situation occurs, nurses must develop a better way of physically restraining patients, taking patients' safety, comfort, and potential adverse outcomes into consideration. Currently, use of a wrist belt tied to the bedside railing is the most common method of restraining patients.

Unplanned extubation usually occurs when a patient moves his or her hand to reach and pull out the tube. A 30° elevation of the head of the bed is common to avoid aspiration and promote ventilation[21]; however, such elevation increases the chance of unplanned extubation. Researchers have suggested that a patient's hands should be kept at least 20 cm away from the tubes,[22] and avoiding the head-up position might prevent unplanned extubation.[23] More investigations are needed to develop better appliances and methods for physical restraint.

Clinical Implications

The Figure summarizes the risk of unplanned extubation. These results may help remind nurses about the risks involved when physical restraints are used in the ICU. The precautions against unplanned extubation begin when a patient is admitted to the other reason requires careful evaluation, because use of physical restraint increases the risk for unplanned extubation by 3.11 times, and the risk increases to 12.44 times if a nosocomial infection is also present. Without physical restraints, the risk of unplanned extubation in a patient with a GCS score of 9 or greater on ICU admission who has an infection is only 4.00 times greater than the risk in a patient with a GCS score less than 9 and no nosocomial infection. In our study, patients with an infection had a higher risk (odds ratio, 2.71; 95% confidence interval, 1.29-5.65) of being restrained [Table 2]. Caution is needed when the use of physical restraint is being considered. Initiation of physical restraint on a patient with an infection will increase the risk of unplanned extubation up to 6.28 times, which is much higher than the risk of unplanned extubation in a patient with only an infection (2.02 times).

Limitation of the Study

In this study, data were obtained by reviewing the medical charts and incident reports. We assumed that the data were documented accurately and adequately. Our findings may be biased because of selective deposit and selective survival, which are common in studies that use existing data. Therefore, further investigation is necessary.

Conclusions

A GCS score of 9 or greater on ICU admission increases the risk of unplanned extubation. Patients are more likely to have an unplanned extubation when they are physically restrained. The risk becomes higher in the presence of nosocomial infection. To minimize the risk of unplanned extubation, nurses must assess patients' GCS status and evaluate the risk of applying physical restraint. To promote patients' safety, we must develop effective standards for use of physical restraints so that we can prevent unplanned extubation.

Acknowledgments Appreciation is extended to all the participating administrators, staff, and patients at the Taichung Veterans General Hospital whose support made this study possible.

Financial Disclosures This research was supported by grants from the Taichung Veterans General Hospital Research Program (TCVGH-917412A).

References

1. Birkett KM, Southerland KA, Leslie GD. Reporting unplanned extubation. *Intensive Crit Care Nurs.* 2005;21(2):65-75.

2. Pandey CK, Singh N, Srivastava K, et al. Self-extubation in intensive care and re-intubation predictors: a retrospective study. *J Indian Med Assoc.* 2002;100(1):11,14-16.

3. Yeh S, Lee L, Ho T, Chiang M, Lin L. Implications of nursing care in the occurrence and consequences of unplanned extubation in adult ICUs. *Int J Nurs Stud.* 2004;41(3):255-262.

4. Happ MB. Treatment interference in critically ill patients: an update on unplanned extubation. *Clin Pulmon Med.* 2002; 9:81-86.

5. Abrahamsen C. Patient restraints: JCAHO and HCFA issue new restraint guidelines. *Nurs Manage.* 2001;32:69-70.

6. De Lassence A, Alberti C, Azoulay E, et al. Impact of unplanned extubation and reintubation after weaning on nosocomial pneumonia risk in the ICU. *Anesthesiology.* 2002;97(1):148-156.

7. Boulain T, Association des Réanimateurs du Centre-Ouest. Unplanned extubations in the adult intensive care unit: prospective multicenter study. *Am J Respir Crit Care Med.* 1998;157(4 pt 1):1131-1137.

8. Krayem A, Butler R, Martin C. Unplanned extubation in the ICU: impact on outcome and nursing workload. *Ann Thorac Med.* 2006;1:71-75.

9. Christie JM, Dethlefsen M, Cane RD. Unplanned endotracheal extubation in the ICU. *J Clin Anesth.* 1996;8(4):289-293.

10. Phoa LL, Pek WY, Syap W, Johan A. Unplanned extubation: a local experience. *Singapore Med J.* 2002;43(10):504-508.

11. Razek T, Gracias V, Sullivan D, et al. Assessing the need for reintubation: a prospective evaluation of unplanned endotracheal extubation. *J Trauma.* 2000;48(3):466-469.

12. Krinsley JS, Barone JE. The drive to survive: unplanned extubation in the ICU. *Chest.* 2005; 128(2):560-566.

13. Chen CZ, Chu YC, Lee CH, Chen CW, Chang HY, Hsiue TR. Factors predicting reintubation after unplanned extubation. *J Formos Med Assoc.* 2002;101(8):542-546.

14. Mort TC. Unplanned tracheal extubation outside the operating room: a quality improvement audit of hemodynamic and tracheal airway complications associated with emergency tracheal reintubation. *Anesth Analg.* 1998:86(6): 1171-1176.

15. Pesiri AJ, Stewart K, Kobe E, Stewart W. Protocol for prevention of unintentional extubation. *Crit Care Nurs Q.* 1990;12(4):87-90.

16. Tominaga GT, Rudzwick H, Scannell G, Waxman K. Decreasing unplanned extubations in the surgical ICU. *Am J Surg.* 1995; 170(6): 586-590.

17. Chevron V, Menard JF, Richard JC, Girault C, Leroy J, Bonmarchand G. Unplanned extubation: risk factors of development and predictive criteria for reintubation. *Crit Care Med.* 1998; 26(6):1049-1053.

18. Balon JA. Common factors of spontaneous self-extubation in a critical care setting. *Int J Trauma Nurs.* 2001;7(3):93-99.

19. Fletcher RH, Fletcher SW, Wagner EH. *Clinical Epidemiology: The Essentials.* 3rd ed. Baltimore, MD: Williams & Wilkins; 1996.

20. Horan TC, Gaynes RP. Surveillance of nosocomial infections. In: Mayhall CG, ed. *Hospital Epidemiology and Infection Control.* 3rd ed. Philadelphia, PA: Lippincott Williams & Wilkins; 2004:1659-1702.

21. Chastre J, Fagon J. Ventilator-associated pneumonia. *Am J Respir Crit Care Med.* 2002;165(7): 867-903.

22. Carrión MI, Ayuso D, Marcos M, et al. Accidental removal of endotracheal and nasogastric tubes and intravascular catheters. *Crit Care Med.* 2000;28(1): 63-66.

23. Grap MJ, Glass C, Lindamood MO. Factors related to unplanned extubation of endotracheal tubes. *Crit Care Nurse.* 1995;15(2):57-65.

APPENDIX B REVIEW QUESTIONS

1. The title of the article tells you right away about the study design. What is it, and what do you know this means?

   _____

   _____

2. What are the advantages and disadvantages of this type of study?

   _____

   _____

3. What is the outcome that the researchers are interested in examining?

   _____

   _____

4. Why is the outcome of interest a concern, and how do the researchers use statistics to make this argument meaningful?

   _____

   _____

5. What is the "exposure" they want to examine?

   _____

   _____

6. How do the nurse researchers use statistics to indicate a need to examine this exposure?

   _____

   _____

7. Look at the methods section of the article, which includes more information about the design and sample used by this research team. Where was the study sample collected?

   _____

   _____

8. Would you anticipate this study population to be representative of the general population in the United States? Why or why not?

   _____

   _____

(continues)

9. What type of study sample was involved in this research?

_____

_____

10. How does the sampling technique limit the application of the results?

_____

_____

11. Who were the cases in study? Who were the controls?

_____

_____

12. In the data analysis portion of the article, the authors report that they completed a power analysis to determine the power of their study with the sample size utilized. They report a power of 90%. What does this mean? Is it adequate?

_____

_____

13. If the power is 90%, what is the likelihood of making a type two error?

_____

_____

14. The researchers also state that they used an alpha of 0.05. What does this mean?

_____

_____

15. What is the null hypothesis for this study?

_____

_____

16. The results section of the article begins with something you may find confusing. Remember that case control studies do not give you incidence data. What are incidence cases?

_____

_____

17. The results section begins by telling you that the incidence rate for unplanned extubations is 8.7%. Why can this study report incidence rates for unplanned extubations?

_____

_____

18. Is the incident rate for unplanned extubations in this study consistent with the ranges reported in the other studies cited in the literature review?

_____

_____

19. What was the average length of time for mechanical ventilation before unplanned extubation?

_____

_____

20. What was the mean score on the Glasgow Coma Scale (GCS) when unplanned extubations occurred?

_____

_____

21. What percentage of unplanned extubations occurred after day one but still within the first week of mechanical ventilation?

_____

_____

22. What percentage of the patients who were reintubated were reintubated within the first hour?

_____

_____

23. The researchers used a *t*-test to examine the mean GCS scores on admission for the unplanned extubation group and the controls. What was the mean score for each group? Which group had higher scores? Were they significantly different?

_____

_____

(continues)

24. Was there a significant difference in the length of ICU stay for the two groups?

_____

_____

25. The authors of the study now move on to a subanalysis within their study, focusing on those who were restrained and those who were not. They divide the 300 subjects in the study based on whether they were restrained or not (this is another case control design). Then they look back to determine whether they had any differing characteristics that may have affected the decision on and the consequences of restraints. What differences did they find in those who were restrained versus those who were not? Were these differences significant?

_____

_____

26. The authors use the chi-square test to see whether there is a difference in the type of intubation (nasal or oral) and in the use of physical restraints (yes or no). What level of measurement are these two variables? What test would be appropriate to determine whether there is a significant difference in the groups? If the associated p-value is 0.46, is there a significant difference between the two groups?

_____

_____

27. The authors report that the mean number of days intubated for those who were physically restrained is 16.8 and that the mean number of days for those who were not was 14.9. What would be an appropriate test to determine whether the difference between the two groups is significant?

_____

_____

28. A chi-square test was run to determine whether there was a difference in gender between those who were and those who were not restrained. The results are chi-square $= 1.93, p = 0.16$. Was there a significant difference?

_____

_____

29. The authors examine the group that was restrained compared to the group that was not and report an odds ratio (OR) of 2.71 (95% CI 1.29–5.65) for nosocomial infection. What does this mean?

_____

_____

30. Within the group of patients who were physically restrained, the authors then examine the patients with unplanned extubation compared to those without unplanned extubation. They looked for differences other than physical restraints that may have contributed to the unplanned extubation. Did they find any significant differences?

_____

_____

31. The authors then look at the group that wasn't restrained and compare patients with and those without unplanned extubation to identify other factors that may contribute to unplanned extubations when no restraints are used. Did they find any significant differences?

_____

_____

32. The authors proceed to a technique you will learn in future statistics classes, which involves a procedure called regression. To use this procedure correctly, you must first identify variables that appear to have a significant effect on your outcome. The authors did so in the previous analyses and chose to examine the effect of the three differences they found on the outcome of unplanned extubations. What were the three variables they believe are associated with unplanned extubations?

_____

_____

33. Why didn't they include age as a variable?

_____

_____

(continues)

34. The nurse researchers determine that using a GCS score of 9 as a predictor of unplanned extubation has a sensitivity of 85% and a specificity of 80.8%. What does this mean?

_____

_____

35. When the authors determined that the relative risk for a patient with a GCS of 9 or over was 1.98. What does this mean statistically and in English?

_____

_____

36. What happens to the RR for unplanned extubation when a patient with a GCS score over 9 is then restrained?

_____

_____

37. What happens to the RR for unplanned extubation when a patient with a GCS score of 9 is restrained and then develops a nosocomial infection?

_____

_____

38. Why might these results be clinically significant?

_____

_____

ANSWERS TO APPENDIX B REVIEW QUESTIONS

1. This is a case control study. The researchers select a group of people who have the outcome of interest and look back to determine what exposures they may have had. They then compare this to a group of individuals who did not have the outcome of interest and the exposures that that group had.

3. Unplanned extubation

5. Use of physical restraints

7. In a 42-bed open-room setting adult ICU at Taichung Veterans General Hospital in Taiwan, China.

9. Nonprobability convenience sample, which included all patients who were admitted and intubated in the ICU during a 21-month period.

11. From the study population, 100 patients with unplanned extubation were selected as cases and compared to 200 matched patients (controls) who were ventilated but did not have an unplanned extubation.

13. $100\% - 90\% = 10\%$ chance of making a type two error

15. H_0: There is no difference in the number of unplanned extubations between patients who have physical restraints and those who do not have physical restraints.

17. This study is actually called a nested case control study, that is, a case control study within a cohort study. Just when you think you understand something, research always seems to throw you a curve!

   The case control study draws data from a cohort of individuals who arrived on an ICU unit intubated and selected those who had unplanned extubations and compared them to controls who didn't. Then the study looked back to determine whether they were physically restrained at the time of the unplanned extubation.

   However, the original study population was a cohort. The number of those patients who then experienced an unplanned extubation is the number of new unplanned extubations during the time of study, which is incidence data. The researchers are now reporting rates from the whole population from which the sample was drawn, which consists of the 1455 patients admitted during the 21-month period. They have data from these patients when they first arrived on the unit intubated and report how many experience an unplanned extubation. This is the incidence rate for unplanned extubation.

19. Mean = 8.6 days

(continues)

21. Cumulative percentage for first week (54%) − Percentage extubated on first day (14%) = 40%

23. Mean for cases = 10.1

    Mean for controls = 9.2

    The scores were higher (better) for the cases (those with unplanned extubations) and were significantly different ($p = 0.002$).

25. Those who were restrained had:
        Higher GCS scores on admission ($p < 0.001$ = significant).
        Higher rates of nosocomial infection ($p = 0.005$ = significant).
        Higher rates of unplanned extubation ($p < 0.001$ = significant).
        Longer ICU stay ($p = 0.009$ = significant).

27. The *t*-test is appropriate for ratio level outcome data and when you are looking for a difference in means between two independent groups.

29. Statistically speaking, it means that the odds are 2.71 times higher that a patient who is restrained has a nosocomial infection compared to a patient who is not restrained.

    The OR is an estimate of relative risk. This study estimates that individuals who have a nosocomial infection are 2.71 times as likely to have had restraints used.

31. Yes, those with unplanned extubations had higher GCS scores on admission ($p = 0.004$).

33. Age was not significantly associated with unplanned extubations or restraint use. They had already done the analysis to show it wasn't a contributing factor.

35. The relative risk is the incidence rate in the exposed sample (those who have a 9 or higher) divided by the incidence rate in the unexposed sample (those who have less than a 9).

    Intensive care patients with an admission score of 9 or higher on the admission assessment of the GCS are 1.98 times as likely to have an unplanned extubation as those who score below a 9.

37. The RR increases again to 12.44. This group of patients is more than 12 times as likely to experience an unplanned extubation as those without these three risk factors.

Appendix C

Tables for Reference

Table 1 t Table. Table entries are values of t random variables.

Cumulative probability	0.75	0.80	0.85	0.90	0.95	0.975	0.99	0.995	0.9975	0.999	0.9995
Upper-tail probability	0.25	0.20	0.15	0.10	0.05	0.025	0.01	0.005	0.0025	0.001	0.0005
1	1.000	1.376	1.963	3.078	6.314	12.71	31.82	63.66	127.3	318.3	636.6
2	0.816	1.061	1.386	1.886	2.920	4.303	6.965	9.925	14.09	22.33	31.60
3	0.765	0.978	1.250	1.638	2.353	3.182	4.541	5.841	7.453	10.21	12.92
4	0.741	0.941	1.190	1.533	2.132	2.776	3.747	4.604	5.598	7.173	8.610
5	0.727	0.920	1.156	1.476	2.015	2.571	3.365	4.032	4.773	5.893	6.869
6	0.718	0.906	1.134	1.440	1.943	2.447	3.143	3.707	4.317	5.208	5.959
7	0.711	0.896	1.119	1.415	1.895	2.365	2.998	3.499	4.029	4.785	5.408
8	0.706	0.889	1.108	1.397	1.860	2.306	2.896	3.355	3.833	4.501	5.041

degrees of freedom

Table 1 t Table. (continued)

| Cumulative probability | 0.75 | 0.80 | 0.85 | 0.90 | 0.95 | 0.975 | 0.99 | 0.995 | 0.9975 | 0.999 | 0.9995 |
Upper-tail probability	0.25	0.20	0.15	0.10	0.05	0.025	0.01	0.005	0.0025	0.001	0.0005
9	0.703	0.883	1.100	1.383	1.833	2.262	2.821	3.250	3.690	4.297	4.781
10	0.700	0.879	1.093	1.372	1.812	2.228	2.764	3.169	3.581	4.144	4.587
11	0.697	0.876	1.088	1.363	1.796	2.201	2.718	3.106	3.497	4.025	4.437
12	0.695	0.873	1.083	1.356	1.782	2.179	2.681	3.055	3.428	3.930	4.318
13	0.694	0.870	1.079	1.350	1.771	2.160	2.650	3.012	3.372	3.852	4.221
14	0.692	0.868	1.076	1.345	1.761	2.145	2.624	2.977	3.326	3.787	4.140
15	0.691	0.866	1.074	1.341	1.753	2.131	2.602	2.947	3.286	3.733	4.073
16	0.690	0.865	1.071	1.337	1.746	2.120	2.583	2.921	3.252	3.686	4.015
17	0.689	0.863	1.069	1.333	1.740	2.110	2.567	2.898	3.222	3.646	3.965
18	0.688	0.862	1.067	1.330	1.734	2.101	2.552	2.878	3.197	3.610	3.922
19	0.688	0.861	1.066	1.328	1.729	2.093	2.539	2.861	3.174	3.579	3.883
20	0.687	0.860	1.064	1.325	1.725	2.086	2.528	2.845	3.153	3.552	3.850
21	0.686	0.859	1.063	1.323	1.721	2.080	2.518	2.831	3.135	3.527	3.819
22	0.686	0.858	1.061	1.321	1.717	2.074	2.508	2.819	3.119	3.505	3.792
23	0.685	0.858	1.060	1.319	1.714	2.069	2.500	2.807	3.104	3.485	3.768
24	0.685	0.857	1.059	1.318	1.711	2.064	2.492	2.797	3.091	3.467	3.745
25	0.684	0.856	1.058	1.316	1.708	2.060	2.485	2.787	3.078	3.450	3.725
26	0.684	0.856	1.058	1.315	1.706	2.056	2.479	2.779	3.067	3.435	3.707
27	0.684	0.855	1.057	1.314	1.703	2.052	2.473	2.771	3.057	3.421	3.690
28	0.683	0.855	1.056	1.313	1.701	2.048	2.467	2.763	3.047	3.408	3.674
29	0.683	0.854	1.055	1.311	1.699	2.045	2.462	2.756	3.038	3.396	3.659
30	0.683	0.854	1.055	1.310	1.697	2.042	2.457	2.750	3.030	3.385	3.646
40	0.681	0.851	1.050	1.303	1.684	2.021	2.423	2.704	2.971	3.307	3.551
60	0.679	0.848	1.045	1.296	1.671	2.000	2.390	2.660	2.915	3.232	3.460
80	0.678	0.846	1.043	1.292	1.664	1.990	2.374	2.639	2.887	3.195	3.416
100	0.677	0.845	1.042	1.290	1.660	1.984	2.364	2.626	2.871	3.174	3.390
1000	0.675	0.842	1.037	1.282	1.646	1.962	2.330	2.581	2.813	3.098	3.300
z	0.674	0.842	1.036	1.282	1.645	1.960	2.326	2.576	2.807	3.090	3.291
Confidence level	50%	60%	70%	80%	90%	95%	98%	99%	99.5%	99.8%	99.9%

degrees of freedom

t values computed with Microsoft Excel 9.0 TINV function.

Table 2 F table. Table entries are F values with right-tail probability *P*.

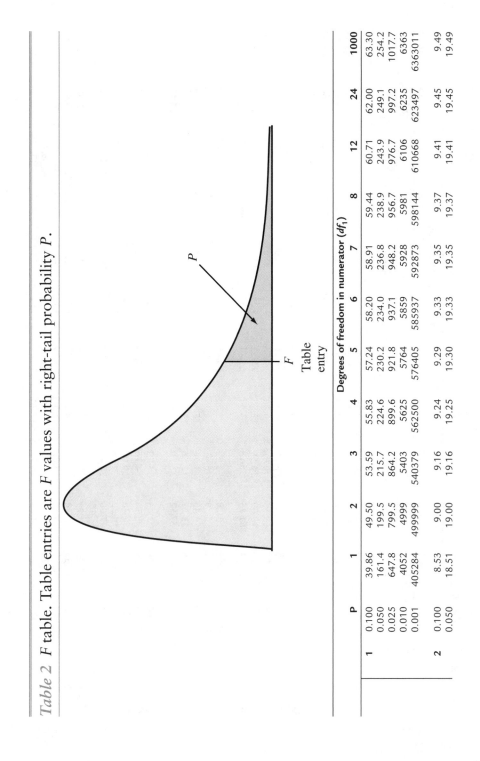

	P	1	2	3	4	5	6	7	8	12	24	1000
1	0.100	39.86	49.50	53.59	55.83	57.24	58.20	58.91	59.44	60.71	62.00	63.30
	0.050	161.4	199.5	215.7	224.6	230.2	234.0	236.8	238.9	243.9	249.1	254.2
	0.025	647.8	799.5	864.2	899.6	921.8	937.1	948.2	956.7	976.7	997.2	1017.7
	0.010	4052	4999	5403	5625	5764	5859	5928	5981	6106	6235	6363
	0.001	405284	499999	540379	562500	576405	585937	592873	598144	610668	623497	6363011
2	0.100	8.53	9.00	9.16	9.24	9.29	9.33	9.35	9.37	9.41	9.45	9.49
	0.050	18.51	19.00	19.16	19.25	19.30	19.33	19.35	19.37	19.41	19.45	19.49

Table 2 F table. *(continued)*

df_2	P	\multicolumn{11}{c}{Degrees of freedom in numerator (df_1)}
		1	2	3	4	5	6	7	8	12	24	1000
2	0.025	38.51	39.00	39.17	39.25	39.30	39.33	39.36	39.37	39.41	39.46	39.50
	0.010	98.50	99.00	99.17	99.25	99.30	99.33	99.36	99.37	99.42	99.46	99.50
	0.001	998.50	999.00	999.17	999.25	999.30	999.33	999.36	999.37	999.42	999.46	999.50
3	0.100	5.54	5.46	5.39	5.34	5.31	5.28	5.27	5.25	5.22	5.18	5.13
	0.050	10.13	9.55	9.28	9.12	9.01	8.94	8.89	8.85	8.74	8.64	8.53
	0.025	17.44	16.04	15.44	15.10	14.88	14.73	14.62	14.54	14.34	14.12	13.91
	0.010	34.12	30.82	29.46	28.71	28.24	27.91	27.67	27.49	27.05	26.60	26.14
	0.001	167.03	148.50	141.11	137.10	134.58	132.85	131.58	130.62	128.32	125.93	123.53
4	0.100	4.54	4.32	4.19	4.11	4.05	4.01	3.98	3.95	3.90	3.83	3.76
	0.050	7.71	6.94	6.59	6.39	6.26	6.16	6.09	6.04	5.91	5.77	5.63
	0.025	12.22	10.65	9.98	9.60	9.36	9.20	9.07	8.98	8.75	8.51	8.26
	0.010	21.20	18.00	16.69	15.98	15.52	15.21	14.98	14.80	14.37	13.93	13.47
	0.001	74.14	61.25	56.18	53.44	51.71	50.53	49.66	49.00	47.41	45.77	44.09
5	0.100	4.06	3.78	3.62	3.52	3.45	3.40	3.37	3.34	3.27	3.19	3.11
	0.050	6.61	5.79	5.41	5.19	5.05	4.95	4.88	4.82	4.68	4.53	4.37
	0.025	10.01	8.43	7.76	7.39	7.15	6.98	6.85	6.76	6.52	6.28	6.02
	0.010	16.26	13.27	12.06	11.39	10.97	10.67	10.46	10.29	9.89	9.47	9.03
	0.001	47.18	37.12	33.20	31.09	29.75	28.83	28.16	27.65	26.42	25.13	23.82
6	0.100	3.78	3.46	3.29	3.18	3.11	3.05	3.01	2.98	2.90	2.82	2.72
	0.050	5.99	5.14	4.76	4.53	4.39	4.28	4.21	4.15	4.00	3.84	3.67
	0.025	8.81	7.26	6.60	6.23	5.99	5.82	5.70	5.60	5.37	5.12	4.86
	0.010	13.75	10.92	9.78	9.15	8.75	8.47	8.26	8.10	7.72	7.31	6.89
	0.001	35.51	27.00	23.70	21.92	20.80	20.03	19.46	19.03	17.99	16.90	15.77
7	0.100	3.59	3.26	3.07	2.96	2.88	2.83	2.78	2.75	2.67	2.58	2.47
	0.050	5.59	4.74	4.35	4.12	3.97	3.87	3.79	3.73	3.57	3.41	3.23
	0.025	8.07	6.54	5.89	5.52	5.29	5.12	4.99	4.90	4.67	4.41	4.15
	0.010	12.25	9.55	8.45	7.85	7.46	7.19	6.99	6.84	6.47	6.07	5.66
	0.001	29.25	21.69	18.77	17.20	16.21	15.52	15.02	14.63	13.71	12.73	11.72

Degrees of freedom in denominator (df_2)

Table 2 F table. *(continued)*

| df_2 | P | \multicolumn{11}{c}{Degrees of freedom in numerator (df_1)} |
		1	2	3	4	5	6	7	8	12	24	1000
8	0.100	3.46	3.11	2.92	2.81	2.73	2.67	2.62	2.59	2.50	2.40	2.30
	0.050	5.32	4.46	4.07	3.84	3.69	3.58	3.50	3.44	3.28	3.12	2.93
	0.025	7.57	6.06	5.42	5.05	4.82	4.65	4.53	4.43	4.20	3.95	3.68
	0.010	11.26	8.65	7.59	7.01	6.63	6.37	6.18	6.03	5.67	5.28	4.87
	0.001	25.41	18.49	15.83	14.39	13.48	12.86	12.40	12.05	11.19	10.30	9.36
9	0.100	3.36	3.01	2.81	2.69	2.61	2.55	2.51	2.47	2.38	2.28	2.16
	0.050	5.12	4.26	3.86	3.63	3.48	3.37	3.29	3.23	3.07	2.90	2.71
	0.025	7.21	5.71	5.08	4.72	4.48	4.32	4.20	4.10	3.87	3.61	3.34
	0.010	10.56	8.02	6.99	6.42	6.06	5.80	5.61	5.47	5.11	4.73	4.32
	0.001	22.86	16.39	13.90	12.56	11.71	11.13	10.70	10.37	9.57	8.72	7.84
10	0.100	3.29	2.92	2.73	2.61	2.52	2.46	2.41	2.38	2.28	2.18	2.06
	0.050	4.96	4.10	3.71	3.48	3.33	3.22	3.14	3.07	2.91	2.74	2.54
	0.025	6.94	5.46	4.83	4.47	4.24	4.07	3.95	3.85	3.62	3.37	3.09
	0.010	10.04	7.56	6.55	5.99	5.64	5.39	5.20	5.06	4.71	4.33	3.92
	0.001	21.04	14.91	12.55	11.28	10.48	9.93	9.52	9.20	8.45	7.64	6.78
12	0.100	3.18	2.81	2.61	2.48	2.39	2.33	2.28	2.24	2.15	2.04	1.91
	0.050	4.75	3.89	3.49	3.26	3.11	3.00	2.91	2.85	2.69	2.51	2.30
	0.025	6.55	5.10	4.47	4.12	3.89	3.73	3.61	3.51	3.28	3.02	2.73
	0.010	9.33	6.93	5.95	5.41	5.06	4.82	4.64	4.50	4.16	3.78	3.37
	0.001	18.64	12.97	10.80	9.63	8.89	8.38	8.00	7.71	7.00	6.25	5.44
14	0.100	3.10	2.73	2.52	2.39	2.31	2.24	2.19	2.15	2.05	1.94	1.80
	0.050	4.60	3.74	3.34	3.11	2.96	2.85	2.76	2.70	2.53	2.35	2.14
	0.025	6.30	4.86	4.24	3.89	3.66	3.50	3.38	3.29	3.05	2.79	2.50
	0.010	8.86	6.51	5.56	5.04	4.69	4.46	4.28	4.14	3.80	3.43	3.02
	0.001	17.14	11.78	9.73	8.62	7.92	7.44	7.08	6.80	6.13	5.41	4.62
16	0.100	3.05	2.67	2.46	2.33	2.24	2.18	2.13	2.09	1.99	1.87	1.72
	0.050	4.49	3.63	3.24	3.01	2.85	2.74	2.66	2.59	2.42	2.24	2.02
	0.025	6.12	4.69	4.08	3.73	3.50	3.34	3.22	3.12	2.89	2.63	2.32
	0.010	8.53	6.23	5.29	4.77	4.44	4.20	4.03	3.89	3.55	3.18	2.76
	0.001	16.12	10.97	9.01	7.94	7.27	6.80	6.46	6.19	5.55	4.85	4.08
18	0.100	3.01	2.62	2.42	2.29	2.20	2.13	2.08	2.04	1.93	1.81	1.66
	0.050	4.41	3.55	3.16	2.93	2.77	2.66	2.58	2.51	2.34	2.15	1.92
	0.025	5.98	4.56	3.95	3.61	3.38	3.22	3.10	3.01	2.77	2.50	2.20

Degrees of freedom in denominator (df_2)

Table 2 F table. *(continued)*

	P	1	2	3	4	5	6	7	8	12	24	1000
18	0.010	8.29	6.01	5.09	4.58	4.25	4.01	3.84	3.71	3.37	3.00	2.58
	0.001	15.38	10.39	8.49	7.46	6.81	6.35	6.02	5.76	5.13	4.45	3.69
20	0.100	2.97	2.59	2.38	2.25	2.16	2.09	2.04	2.00	1.89	1.77	1.61
	0.050	4.35	3.49	3.10	2.87	2.71	2.60	2.51	2.45	2.28	2.08	1.85
	0.025	5.87	4.46	3.86	3.51	3.29	3.13	3.01	2.91	2.68	2.41	2.09
	0.010	8.10	5.85	4.94	4.43	4.10	3.87	3.70	3.56	3.23	2.86	2.43
	0.001	14.82	9.95	8.10	7.10	6.46	6.02	5.69	5.44	4.82	4.15	3.40
30	0.100	2.88	2.49	2.28	2.14	2.05	1.98	1.93	1.88	1.77	1.64	1.46
	0.050	4.17	3.32	2.92	2.69	2.53	2.42	2.33	2.27	2.09	1.89	1.63
	0.025	5.57	4.18	3.59	3.25	3.03	2.87	2.75	2.65	2.41	2.14	1.80
	0.010	7.56	5.39	4.51	4.02	3.70	3.47	3.30	3.17	2.84	2.47	2.02
	0.001	13.29	8.77	7.05	6.12	5.53	5.12	4.82	4.58	4.00	3.36	2.61
50	0.100	2.81	2.41	2.20	2.06	1.97	1.90	1.84	1.80	1.68	1.54	1.33
	0.050	4.03	3.18	2.79	2.56	2.40	2.29	2.20	2.13	1.95	1.74	1.45
	0.025	5.34	3.97	3.39	3.05	2.83	2.67	2.55	2.46	2.22	1.93	1.56
	0.010	7.17	5.06	4.20	3.72	3.41	3.19	3.02	2.89	2.56	2.18	1.70
	0.001	12.22	7.96	6.34	5.46	4.90	4.51	4.22	4.00	3.44	2.82	2.05
100	0.100	2.76	2.36	2.14	2.00	1.91	1.83	1.78	1.73	1.61	1.46	1.22
	0.050	3.94	3.09	2.70	2.46	2.31	2.19	2.10	2.03	1.85	1.63	1.30
	0.025	5.18	3.83	3.25	2.92	2.70	2.54	2.42	2.32	2.08	1.78	1.36
	0.010	6.90	4.82	3.98	3.51	3.21	2.99	2.82	2.69	2.37	1.98	1.45
	0.001	11.50	7.41	5.86	5.02	4.48	4.11	3.83	3.61	3.07	2.46	1.64
1000	0.100	2.71	2.31	2.09	1.95	1.85	1.78	1.72	1.68	1.55	1.39	1.08
	0.050	3.85	3.00	2.61	2.38	2.22	2.11	2.02	1.95	1.76	1.53	1.11
	0.025	5.04	3.70	3.13	2.80	2.58	2.42	2.30	2.20	1.96	1.65	1.13
	0.010	6.66	4.63	3.80	3.34	3.04	2.82	2.66	2.53	2.20	1.81	1.16
	0.001	10.89	6.96	5.46	4.65	4.14	3.78	3.51	3.30	2.77	2.16	1.22

Degrees of freedom in numerator (df_1)

Degrees of freedom in denominator (df_2)

Note: F values computed with Microsoft Excel 9.0 FINV function.

Table 3 Chi-square table.

Table entries are chi-square values
with right-tail probability *P*.

df	0.975	0.25	0.20	0.15	0.10	0.05	0.025	0.01	0.005	0.001	0.0005
1	0.00098	1.32	1.64	2.07	2.71	3.84	5.02	6.63	7.88	10.83	12.12
2	0.051	2.77	3.22	3.79	4.61	5.99	7.38	9.21	10.60	13.82	15.20
3	0.216	4.11	4.64	5.32	6.25	7.81	9.35	11.34	12.84	16.27	17.73
4	0.48	5.39	5.99	6.74	7.78	9.49	11.14	13.28	14.86	18.47	20.00
5	0.83	6.63	7.29	8.12	9.24	11.07	12.83	15.09	16.75	20.52	22.11
6	1.24	7.84	8.56	9.45	10.64	12.59	14.45	16.81	18.55	22.46	24.10
7	1.69	9.04	9.80	10.75	12.02	14.07	16.01	18.48	20.28	24.32	26.02
8	2.18	10.22	11.03	12.03	13.36	15.51	17.53	20.09	21.95	26.12	27.87
9	2.70	11.39	12.24	13.29	14.68	16.92	19.02	21.67	23.59	27.88	29.67
10	3.25	12.55	13.44	14.53	15.99	18.31	20.48	23.21	25.19	29.59	31.42
11	3.82	13.70	14.63	15.77	17.28	19.68	21.92	24.72	26.76	31.26	33.14
12	4.40	14.85	15.81	16.99	18.55	21.03	23.34	26.22	28.30	32.91	34.82
13	5.01	15.98	16.98	18.20	19.81	22.36	24.74	27.69	29.82	34.53	36.48
14	5.63	17.12	18.15	19.41	21.06	23.68	26.12	29.14	31.32	36.12	38.11
15	6.26	18.25	19.31	20.60	22.31	25.00	27.49	30.58	32.80	37.70	39.72

Table 3 Chi-square table. *(continued)*

df	0.975	0.25	0.20	0.15	0.10	0.05	0.025	0.01	0.005	0.001	0.0005
						Probability in right tail					
16	6.91	19.37	20.47	21.79	23.54	26.30	28.85	32.00	34.27	39.25	41.31
17	7.56	20.49	21.61	22.98	24.77	27.59	30.19	33.41	35.72	40.79	42.88
18	8.23	21.60	22.76	24.16	25.99	28.87	31.53	34.81	37.16	42.31	44.43
19	8.91	22.72	23.90	25.33	27.20	30.14	32.85	36.19	38.58	43.82	45.97
20	9.59	23.83	25.04	26.50	28.41	31.41	34.17	37.57	40.00	45.31	47.50
21	10.28	24.93	26.17	27.66	29.62	32.67	35.48	38.93	41.40	46.80	49.01
22	10.98	26.04	27.30	28.82	30.81	33.92	36.78	40.29	42.80	48.27	50.51
23	11.69	27.14	28.43	29.98	32.01	35.17	38.08	41.64	44.18	49.73	52.00
24	12.40	28.24	29.55	31.13	33.20	36.42	39.36	42.98	45.56	51.18	53.48
25	13.12	29.34	30.68	32.28	34.38	37.65	40.65	44.31	46.93	52.62	54.95
26	13.84	30.43	31.79	33.43	35.56	38.89	41.92	45.64	48.29	54.05	56.41
27	14.57	31.53	32.91	34.57	36.74	40.11	43.19	46.96	49.64	55.48	57.86
28	15.31	32.62	34.03	35.71	37.92	41.34	44.46	48.28	50.99	56.89	59.30
29	16.05	33.71	35.14	36.85	39.09	42.56	45.72	49.59	52.34	58.30	59.30
30	16.79	34.80	36.25	37.99	40.26	43.8	47.0	50.9	53.7	59.7	62.2
40	24.43	45.62	47.27	49.24	51.81	55.76	59.34	63.69	66.77	73.40	76.09
50	32.36	56.33	58.16	60.35	63.17	67.50	71.42	76.15	79.49	86.66	89.56
60	40.48	66.98	68.97	71.34	74.40	79.08	83.30	88.38	91.95	99.61	102.69
80	57.15	88.13	90.41	93.11	96.58	101.88	106.63	112.33	116.32	124.84	128.26
100	74.22	109.1	111.7	114.7	118.5	124.3	129.6	135.8	140.2	149.4	153.2

Note: Chi-square values computed with Microsoft Excel 9.0 CHINV function.

Index

237